Not Part of the Job

Not Part of the Job

How to Take a Stand Against Violence in the Work Setting

Jane Lipscomb, PhD, RN, FAAN

Matt London, MS

American Nurses Association
Silver Spring, Maryland • 2015

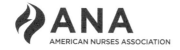

American Nurses Association
8515 Georgia Avenue, Suite 400
Silver Spring, MD 20910-3492
1-800-274-4ANA
www.NursingWorld.org

The American Nurses Association (ANA) is the premier organization representing the interests of the nation's 3.6 million registered nurses. ANA advances the nursing profession by fostering high standards of nursing pratice, promoting a safe and ethical work environment, bolstering the health and wellness of nurses, and advocating on health care issues that affect nurses and the public. ANA is at the forefront of improving the quality of health care for all.

Library of Congress Cataloging-in-Publication Data available upon request.

978-1-55810-595-9   SAN: 851-3481   02/2017R

First printing: March 2015. Second printing: February 2017.

The authors would like to acknowledge the hard work, guidance, and support of many co-workers, especially Kathleen McPhaul, Jonathan Rosen, Janet Foley.

Additionally, this book is dedicated to the nurses and healthcare workers who, on a daily basis, provide compassionate care to their patients, often under the most challenging and, regretably, dangerous conditions.

All healthcare workers, and their patients, deserve a safe environment.

Contents

About the Authors

JANE LIPSCOMB, PHD, RN, FAAN, is a professor at the University of Maryland's Schools of Nursing and Medicine and the Director of the Center for Community-Based Engagement and Learning (CBEL) at the University of Maryland, Baltimore. She has conducted research into the prevention of occupational injuries and illness in the health care and social service workplace for over twenty years, with a focus on workplace violence prevention. Between 1999 and 2012, Dr. Lipscomb and colleagues were awarded four large multi-year grants from the Centers for Disease Control and Prevention and the National Institute for Occupational Safety and Health (NIOSH) to evaluate the impact of a range of risk factors and interventions designed to reduce violence in health care and social service settings.

Prior to joining the faculty, Dr. Lipscomb spent three years as a senior scientist and liaison to the Occupational Safety and Health Administration (OSHA) in the Office of the Director of NIOSH, and five years at the University of California at San Francisco (UCSF) School of Nursing, as Assistant Professor and Director of the graduate program in Occupational Health Nursing. Dr. Lipscomb received her BSN from Boston College, her MS in Occupational Health from Boston University/Harvard School of Public Health, and PhD in Epidemiology from the University of California, Berkeley. Dr. Lipscomb is the recipient of the University of Maryland's 2008 Founders Day Research Lecturer Award. In 1999, she was elected as a Fellow Member of the American Academy of Nursing (FAAN) and in 2013 as Fellow of the Collegium Ramazzini.

MATT LONDON, MS, currently works as a consultant in occupational health and safety, utilizing his training in industrial hygiene and epidemiology and his varied experience as a health and safety professional. He is also currently an adjunct professor in the Department of Family and Community Health at the University of Maryland School of Nursing, as well as the East Coast Coordinator for the Occupational Health Internship Program (OHIP), a nine-week summer health and safety internship program that places undergraduate and graduate students with labor and community organizations.

Matt has also worked as a Health and Safety Specialist for the New York State Public Employees Federation (PEF), a public sector union that represents 54,000 state government workers, including 8,000 nurses. While there, he was PEF's Workplace Violence Prevention Coordinator and served as project coordinator on two five-year CDC-funded participative research projects on workplace violence prevention in state government agencies conducted in conjunction with the University of Maryland. Previously, Matt worked for the New York State Department of Health where he was the Chief of Industrial Hygiene Services and where he developed and coordinated a statewide occupational health clinic network. Earlier, Matt worked in the Hazard Evaluation and Technical Assistance Branch of the National Institute for Occupational Safety and Health (NIOSH), where he designed and implemented study protocols nationwide for a range of occupational health research problems.

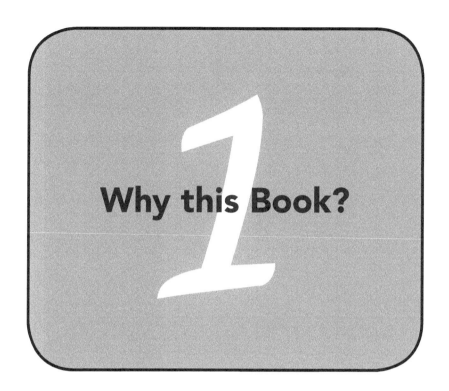

Why this Book?

VIOLENCE TOWARD STAFF IS WIDESPREAD in healthcare and social assistance workplaces, despite decades of attention to the problem by individuals and organizations within the fields of mental health, public health, and nursing. The problem of workplace violence in healthcare and social assistance workplaces continues in part because of a strong reluctance to fully acknowledge and address the problem. A primary factor in this reluctance is the fear of stigmatizing the potential perpetrators of the violence, particularly the mentally ill, developmentally disabled, and cognitively impaired elderly. In addition, healthcare workers and employers often use the question of perpetrator's intent as a reason for not labeling the behavior as violent and therefore not searching for and adopting preventive measures. Unfortunately, there also remains a prevalent attitude that violence toward those working with the public, especially individuals with cognitive impairment, mental illness, or brain injury is part of the job.

Throughout this book, we will discuss this and other factors that create barriers to efforts to reduce violence toward healthcare workers across a range of healthcare and social service settings. We will also offer strategies and tools which we have found effective in addressing and reducing these barriers. While we will offer steps that individual workers can take to make themselves safer while at work, much of our focus is on the critical importance of collective action and building partnerships among workers, patient advocates, administrators, security personnel, and others in order to effect change at the organizational level.

A quick, basic online search of the U.S. National Library of Medicine's PubMed database for papers published in 2013 on the topic "workplace violence" yielded 120 articles. Most describe the problem and discuss risk factors for staff assaults. Many of them infer solutions based on the identification of these risk factors and, of course, all of them call for more research (including papers we ourselves have authored). What is often missing is the frank discussion of why the problem continues and what can be done to mitigate or eliminate this significant cause of worker injury. Our goal in writing this book is to stimulate that conversation and to provide the reader with a primer that will live up to the title of the book *Not Part of the Job: How to Take a Stand Against Violence in the Work Setting.*

In the following pages we will draw upon more than 15 years of field research into workplace violence prevention that we have conducted with partners across four U.S. states (Idaho, Maryland, New York, Washington), as well as our workplace violence prevention consultations with the U.S. Veteran's Health Administration (VHA), the National Institute for Occupational Safety and Health (NIOSH), and the University of West Indies in Kingston, Jamaica. In each project, we worked closely with multiple stakeholders to develop, implement, and evaluate workplace violence prevention programs.

Much of our work was conducted in New York State (NYS) government workplaces. A series of tragic workplace murders in the 1990s led, in part, to enhanced interest in workplace violence prevention on the part of the leading public sector unions and many agency managers in NYS.

With the assistance of research funding from CDC/NIOSH, we were able to conduct participatory action research around workplace violence prevention within a variety of NYS agencies, including five large state-run psychiatric facilities, as well as 13 state-run residential alcohol and substance abuse treatment facilities (Lipscomb et al., 2006; Lipscomb et al., 2012; McPhaul et al., 2008). Across the four states, we conducted more than 50 focus groups on various aspects of workplace violence prevention among direct care staff working in a range of healthcare and social assistance workplaces. Across these four geographically diverse states and across settings within each state we heard many of the same stories and themes. In this book, we share these stories and offer the most important lessons we have learned over these 15 years of work. We will frame these lessons within the context of worker rights and protections to give you the tools so you can take a stand against workplace violence in your workplace, within your professional organization, and at the policy level. Finally, we provide advocacy and research tools that we have developed and used over time to stop the violence in workplaces.

Most of the best practices and case studies we present come from our field experience in public sector agency settings, including psychiatric hospitals, institutional and community settings for the developmentally disabled and mentally retarded, residential addiction treatment centers, juvenile and adult justice facilities, and community mental health settings. We believe that these practices are relevant and transferable to most settings in which you practice.

This book is intended for nurses, other healthcare and social assistance workers, healthcare administrators, professional organizations and unions, and others who have a role or stake in preventing workplace violence. This book is intended as a "how to" manual or primer, not a textbook or summary of the research. We sincerely hope that you will find that the information in these pages helps you reduce workplace violence in your work setting.

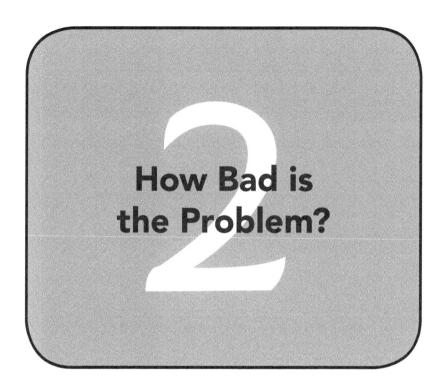

How Bad is the Problem?

SPEAKING AT A PRESS CONFERENCE a few years ago, Jill, a registered nurse at a state-run psychiatric center, said she loves her job despite being hospitalized after an attack in November 1996.

The perpetrator of this attack, a new patient transferred to her care unit, was a 6-foot, 250-pound man with a history of arson who had murdered a woman during a home invasion. Jill said it was not unusual for the center to accept patients with criminal backgrounds.

On that day in 1996, the new patient attempted to strangle Jill by pinning her against a wall, but as she struggled, he changed tactics and began punching her in the face, causing her head to bang against the wall with each blow. She fell to the ground after being pummeled, and he began to kick her repeatedly. "No doubt in my mind I'd be dead," said Jill, but fortunately another patient had overheard the attack and intervened to save her life.

She described the day she left the hospital, including her trip to the police station where she was hunched over in pain and had to support her jaw just so she could talk to authorities. Jill said the police officer at the front desk would not take her statement, telling Jill "you knew the risks before taking the job." The officer took a statement only after Jill's husband's insistence.

Jill's personal account of her assault is unfortunately all too common. Workplace violence is one of the most dangerous occupational hazards facing workers in the healthcare and social assistance sectors. Yet, there is a persistent lack of awareness of the frequency and severity of workers' injuries from patient-related violence, as well as an ignorance of the impact that those assaults have on the workers, their families, co-workers, and even the patients themselves.

Patient/client safety is seen as a priority within healthcare and social services. However, it is often viewed as being separate from, and even in opposition to, staff safety, rather than being understood as being integrally related. This manifests itself in at least a couple of ways. Many of the relevant certifying and/or licensing bodies, e.g., Departments of Health and The Joint Commission (TJC), as well as healthcare administrators, middle managers, and patient advocacy groups prioritize patient safety over worker safety.

In addition, there remains a prevalent attitude that increased risk of violence for those working with individuals with cognitive impairment, mental illness, or brain injury is part of the job. Evidence of this comes from a qualitative study recently published in the Journal of Emergency Nursing which described a culture of acceptance of violence among hospital administrators, prosecutors and judges (Wolf, Delao & Perhats 2014). One emergency nurse assault victim reported being told by a judge: "[W]ell, isn't that the nature of the beast, being in an emergency room and all?" Another told the researchers, "[A]dministration will only take action when some lethal event happens."

Thus, efforts to apply a public health framework which focuses on identifying and addressing upstream factors to reduce the hazard have been limited, even at a time when there is increased recognition of the value of addressing violence in our society in general through a public health framework, including a recent TedTalk on the subject which can be found here: http://www.ted.com/talks/gary_slutkin_let_s_treat_violence_like_a_contagious_disease?utm_

source=newsletter_weekly_2013-10-12&utm_campaign=newsletter_week-
ly&utm_medium=email&utm_content=bottom_right_button.

Our response to the lack of progress in addressing the endemic workplace violence in health care is a call to action to make sure that poli-
cymakers and healthcare administrators understand that the safety of
healthcare workers and the safety of patients are inextricably linked. In
health care, anyone within the facility who has the opportunity for contact
with a potentially violent individual is at risk, including other patients.
In the acute care setting, patients' contact is primarily with healthcare
staff, but those patients also may have contact with other patients and
visitors in non-private rooms, hallways outside patient rooms, the emergency department (ED), and waiting and holding areas. In the community setting, the public-at-large is at risk when an individual with a serious
mental illness destabilizes, as are the nurses, social workers, and others
who dedicate their careers to improving the lives of these often margin-
alized individuals.

When a patient suffers an injury at the hands of another patient (or
staff), the organization may incur legal liability, damaged public relations,
and numerous related costs. The direct costs to the organization resulting
from a healthcare worker injury incurred from a patient assault may
include medical costs and partial wage replacement through the workers'
compensation system, overtime for other staff, potential training and
recruitment of replacement staff. The indirect costs, however, are huge,
and harder to calculate. The quality of patient care suffers when staff
members are injured and unable to work. Lost time injuries may result
in the use of per diem or float staff that may be less familiar with the
unit and patients. In addition, staff members that float to another unit
have been found to experience three times the rate of assaults compared
to staff permanently assigned to their work unit (Hodgson et al., 2004).
Exposure to work-related aggression and violence may also increase the
risk of non-therapeutic or negative responses by staff, ultimately leading
to diminished quality of care. Results from a longitudinal study indicate
that violence experienced by healthcare staff was associated with lower
patient ratings on quality of care (Arnetz & Arnetz, 2001).

The term "workplace violence" is used to describe a range of behaviors
and circumstances across workplaces globally. For the purpose of this
discussion, we use the NIOSH definition: "violent acts, including physical assaults and threats of assault, directed toward persons at work or
on duty" (NIOSH, 1996). Federal OSHA defines workplace violence as

"any act or threat of physical violence, harassment, intimidation, or other threatening disruptive behavior that occurs at the work site" (OSHA, 2014). This definition is preferred by many in nursing because of the explicit inclusion of harassment.

We also discuss workplace violence within the context of the classification scheme published in the 1990s to direct intervention efforts. According to this rubric, workplace violence is classified into four types based on the relationship between the perpetrator and the victim/worker: Type I (Stranger/Criminal Intent), Type II (Customer/Client), Type III (Worker-on-Worker), and Type IV (Personal Relationship) (University of Iowa, 2001). This book focuses primarily on Type II violence but it is our contention that a workplace with endemic patient-on-worker violence is also at increased risk for other types of violence, in part because the organization often does not have a comprehensive violence prevention program that should address all types of workplace violence. Type III violence (worker-on-worker), which includes bullying, is pervasive in the healthcare and social assistance workplace, as well as workplaces in general. Although this book focuses on Type II workplace violence, we have compiled a list of resources on Type III violence (See Appendix A).

What You and Your Employer Should Know About the Problem

THE HAZARD OF WORKPLACE VIOLENCE is well-recognized in the healthcare and social assistance sectors. In 1994, William Charney published the first edition of *Handbook of Hospital Safety* with a chapter dedicated to the hazard of workplace violence (Lipscomb, 1994). In 1996, both NIOSH and OSHA published and broadly disseminated documents describing violence as an occupational hazard in the healthcare workplace, as well as risk factors and prevention strategies for mitigating the hazard (NIOSH, 1996; OSHA, 1996). Later, in 2002, NIOSH published a report entitled *Violence: Occupational Hazards in Hospitals* (NIOSH, 2002). In 2010, The Joint Commission (TJC), an independent, not-for-profit organization that accredits and certifies more than 20,000 U.S. healthcare organizations and programs, issued *Sentinel Event Alert 45: Preventing Violence in the Healthcare Setting* (TJC, 2010).

In recent years, numerous professional associations, including those representing nurses, physicians, psychologists, and social workers have published documents and policy statements addressing workplace violence. In 2008, the American Psychiatric Nurses Association (APNA) published a *Workplace Violence Position Statement* that examined the scope of the problem and identified solutions. Their findings (excerpted below) identified many of the factors we previously addressed in Chapter 1. According to APNA,

> *It is abundantly clear that violence at work from consumers, colleagues, and workplace intruders is a significant occupational health hazard for nurses in all settings. The evidence base is rapidly improving and reports relative to the efficacy of various risk management, regulatory, and legal interventions are identifying important protective measures. Nevertheless, barriers to effectively addressing the problem of workplace violence persist and include inconsistent legal and regulatory protections, widely varying prevention programs lacking an evidence base, the belief that violence is 'part of the work,' and the absence of standardized operational definitions precluding benchmarking and monitoring. (APNA, 2008)*

See Appendix B for recommendations from the report.

The magnitude of the problem of workplace violence in the U.S. is estimated from several national surveys. The first of these is the U.S. Department of Justice National Crime Victimization Survey (NCVS), which for 1993–2009 reported an average of 572,000 "violent victimizations" (e.g. simple and aggravated assaults, rape, sexual assault, robbery) per year that had occurred at work against persons age 16 or older (Harrell, 2011). According to data from this population-based household survey, the overall average annual rate for non-fatal violent crimes at work was estimated to be 5.1 per 1,000. When examined by occupation, the groups within health care with the highest average annual rate of workplace violence were mental health staff (20.5 assaults per 1000 workers) and custodial care workers in mental health (37.6 assaults per 1000 workers).

A second estimate of the size of the problem comes from the U.S. Department of Labor's Bureau of Labor Statistic's (BLS) Annual Survey of Nonfatal Occupational Illness and Injury. According to findings from this survey, health care continues to lead all other industries in the number of nonfatal assaults resulting in lost workdays in the United States, contributing 60% of all such assaults (Bureau of Labor Statistics, 2013).

It should be noted that the BLS survey includes only those injuries that resulted in lost workdays, restricted duty, or medical care beyond first aid and as such, does not capture less severe or non-physical injuries assessed in the NCVS. The BLS survey is considered the primary source of occupational injury and illness data across all workplaces and therefore is an important data source, especially for the purpose of comparing health care with other industries included in the survey. According to the BLS, the rate of nonfatal assaults to workers in the "healthcare and social assistance" industry in 2012 was 15.1 per 10,000 compared to 4.0 per 10,000 in the private sector as a whole (Bureau of Labor Statistics, 2013). This represents an increase from 2011, when the rate in this sector was 14.6 per 10,000 (Bureau of Labor Statistics, 2012).

Pompeii and colleagues (2013) conducted a review of the hospital-based peer reviewed literature (excluding psychiatric hospitals) for the years 2000–2010 for the purpose of estimating the prevalence of workplace violence in this setting. Their review yielded 17 studies, with one-year prevalence ranging from 22%–90% for verbal abuse, 12%–64% for physical threats and 2%–32% for physical assaults reported. They noted that the literature lacked rigorous methods for examining incidents and circumstances surrounding events or rates of events over time.

Another source of data that can be used to measure and track injuries is Workers' Compensation (WC) reports. Nationally and across industry sectors, these data are recognized to seriously undercount workplace injuries and illnesses for a variety of reasons, including that many workers are hesitant to report incidents to their employer or choose to not get involved in the very bureaucratic WC system. Recognizing there are limitations in these data, WC reports are an important source of work-related injury data.

Despite the magnitude of the problem of workplace violence across a range of worksites, high-risk U.S. employers report little attention to workplace violence prevention, even after a violent incident. Over 80% of U.S. employers report "no change" in their workplace violence programming after a significant violent event, even though over 35% of these employers cite negative effects such as absenteeism and reduced productivity in the wake of a violent incident (BLS, 2006).

One cannot discuss the magnitude of the problem of workplace violence in health care without noting that assaults in health care and social assistance have been found to be severely underreported. A study of

76 certified nurse assistants practicing in geriatric settings found that 95% of assaults were not reported (Snyder, Chen, & Vacha-Haase, 2007). Similarly, a study of direct care staff working in two large forensic hospitals in Washington State found 85% of incidents were not reported (Bensley et al., 1997). Research investigating the reasons for not reporting incidents of violence has found such things as the absence of a clear policy regarding reporting (May & Grubbs 2002) and a reticence based on a belief that no action will be taken (Hsiang-Chu & Sheuan, 2011). These, and other related reasons such as fear of retaliation, have been identified in our focus groups and research.

An additional factor in the underreporting of violent incidents is the current emphasis on patient satisfaction and customer service throughout health care. One nurse interviewed as part of a study of underreporting incidents in a large southeastern state reported "[Administration] cares more about patients' perception of our hospital than they do about the staff." Another worker reported,

> If the patient is upset...or acting in an aggressive manner and they say 'I want the supervisor', the supervisor comes down and all of the sudden it's like [the workers] don't matter. Now we have an angry customer and we have to make them happy so they'll give us good marks on our surveys. (Pompeii, APHA presentation, November 19, 2014)

As such, workers are often discouraged from reporting patient behavior for fear of poor satisfaction scores. The following statements came from a nurse manager working in a large healthcare system in a southeastern state:

If we've fought with this patient all the time because we're not giving them morphine, and then the question [on the satisfaction survey] says, 'Was my pain relieved?' that's tied to our [satisfaction] score, which is tied to value-based purchasing, which is the whole of nursing. We're all getting evaluated on that. [Nurse Manager] (Pompeii, APHA presentation, November 19, 2014)

In addition, "Our threats [from patients] now are 'What's your name? Wait until I get my survey.' ... after they yell at you and they curse you out... because they know you are going to get in trouble." (Schoenfisch, APHA presentation, November 19, 2014)

What Do We Know About Risk Factors for Workplace Violence?

WE NOW TURN OUR ATTENTION to what we know about patient, visitor, staff, and work environment factors that contribute to the problem. While discussing these categories of factors, it is important to recognize that it is rarely a single factor but rather the interactions of these factors that contribute to staff (and patient) injury. As such, prevention strategies need to address these factors as they exist in combination within the dynamic healthcare work environment.

The National Institute for Occupational Safety and Health (NIOSH) has identified and published a list of risk factors for workplace violence, including "working with unstable or volatile persons in healthcare, social service, or criminal justice settings" and "working in community-based settings" (NIOSH, 2002) (see Figure 1). Further, the Occupational Safety and Health Administration (OSHA) enumerated additional specific risk factors for those settings, including: the use of hospitals for the care of acutely disturbed, violent individuals; the increased number of mentally ill patients who have been de-institutionalized or released from psychiatric hospitals with inadequate follow-up care; isolated work with clients; lack of staff training; and inadequate staffing during off-shifts and at times of increased activities, such as meal time (OSHA, 2004). These observations by OSHA have been corroborated by our work in multiple settings and locations.

The risk factors for violence vary from hospital to hospital depending on location, size, and type of care. Common risk factors for hospital violence include the following:

- Working directly with volatile people, especially if they are under the influence of drugs or alcohol or have a history of violence or certain psychotic diagnoses
- Working when understaffed—especially during meal times and visiting hours
- Transporting patients
- Long waits for service
- Overcrowded, uncomfortable waiting rooms
- Working alone
- Poor environmental design
- Inadequate security
- Lack of staff training and policies for preventing and managing crises with potentially volatile patients
- Drug and alcohol abuse
- Access to firearms
- Unrestricted movement of the public
- Poorly lit corridors, rooms, parking lots, and other areas

Figure 1. What are the risk factors for violence? (Source: NIOSH, 2002)

PATIENT (PERPETRATOR) CHARACTERISTICS

Much of what is known about individual patient/perpetrator characteristics associated with workplace violence comes from large population-based studies which have primarily focused on subgroups with diagnoses of mental illness and substance abuse disorders. A review of these data suggests that individuals with the following characteristics, in aggregate, pose an increased risk of violence: a history of violent behavior, certain psychotic disorders (schizophrenic spectrum disorders, major affective disorders), substance abuse, dementia, and other conditions limiting cognition and impulse control.

Related to these individual characteristics, it is important to recognize that patients who suffer from mental illness, abuse substances, and/or those who are being seen in the ED often have multiple risk factors in addition to the above that increase their risk for perpetrating violence, including a history of trauma, unemployment, homelessness, and experience in the criminal justice system. In addition, the experience of a traumatic injury and/or physical or mental illness, in combination with an emergency room visit or hospitalization can produce grief, fear, frustration and anxiety and potentially lead to aggression towards staff.

Research examining the relationships among mental health, substance abuse, and violence confirm the fact that most individuals with a mental health diagnosis are not violent. Not all types of psychiatric illness seem to be associated with violence—anxiety disorders, for example, do not seem to increase the risk. However, in the 2006 New England Journal of Medicine editorial titled "Violence and Mental Illness—How Strong is the Link?" R. Friedman cited population-based surveys and reported that patients with schizophrenia, major depression, or bipolar disorder were twice as likely to be assaultive than were people without such an illness. Additionally, the risk associated with a history of substance abuse, was five times the rate of those who had neither condition. Among individuals with major affective disorders and a dual diagnosis of substance abuse, the risk of violence was six times the rate among those who have neither condition. These data highlight the need to counter the stigmatization that often accompanies any person with a major mental health diagnosis, and to focus on the subset of those individuals who do seem to present an increased risk of committing a violent act. Other factors associated with a high risk of violence among psychiatric patients are less clear.

Other research has been published noting that in-patient mental health settings often have a small number of patients who are responsible for a substantial proportion of the patient-on-patient and patient-on-staff assaults. Quanbeck and associates examined data on 839 assaults committed by 88 patients and reported that fellow patients were more likely to be assaulted than staff and the type of assault varied by victim category (2007).

In our work in state-run in-patient psychiatric hospitals, we found that on average, 40%–70% of the patient-on-staff assaults were due to

3–4 patients. The percentages of patient-on-patient assaults committed by just a few patients were similar. These were often, but not always, the same patients.

There were many reported motivations for the assaults by this group of patients, including retaliation, intimidation, sex, and racial differences. Organizational factors that were believed to contribute to assault included rigidity of rules, as well as authoritarian, anxious, or inexperienced staff. Possible prevention strategies included placing repetitively assaultive patients in special treatment units and criminal prosecution of patients with organized and goal-oriented aggression. To our knowledge, research evaluating the impact of such strategies has not been published.

Forensic psychologists, including Doctor Reid Meloy, have also recognized that a small subset of patients seen in psychiatric facilities suffer from psychopathologies for which there may be no effective clinical treatment. Their behavior is predatory in nature; they intend to and do repeatedly harm staff. Direct care workers employed in psychiatric facilities have reported that they recognized these patients but that clinicians were often reluctant to employ other than standard medical protocols to manage these patients, regardless of how many staff they injured.

Compounding the difficulty in predicting violence based on individual patient diagnosis or other clinical characteristics, is a dominant clinician perspective that relies on static patient behavior rather than an assessment of the dynamic and interrelated patient, staff and environmental factors.

FAMILY/VISITOR RISK

Patients are not the only perpetrators of violence directed at workers in the healthcare setting. Family and friends of patients as well as acquaintances may also pose a risk to staff. "Uncertainty, grief, and frustration experienced by patients' family members and friends can translate to physical or verbal aggression toward staff members, patients, or others" (ECRI, 2011). An example of this was the highly publicized 2010 incident at Johns Hopkins Hospital in Baltimore, Maryland, where a family member shot a physician after the physician informed him of his mother's deteriorating medical condition. The man then barricaded himself and his mother in her hospital room, later shooting the mother before turning the gun on himself. Such dramatic incidents are fortunately rare, but this illustrates the potential risk that could apply to anyone with patient interactions in health care.

Visitors may also pose a serious risk to ED personnel when a patient is seeking care for violence-related injuries. Trauma center staff are at risk of violence from gang members who may follow the patient to the ED to retaliate or even attempt murder. We provided consultation on workplace violence to colleagues working in Kingston General Hospital, Jamaica, and learned that this type of activity was a major staff concern and risk factor for assault. Similarly, this problem was raised in focus groups we conducted in multiple states and settings in the U.S. Additionally, patients who present to the hospital ED because they have been injured by their spouse or partner, may pose a risk of workplace violence if the spouse/partner follows the patient to the healthcare facility and causes a violent episode.

STAFF (VICTIM) CHARACTERISTICS

A discussion of individual staff characteristics (e.g. gender, age, or physical stature) associated with workplace assaults is complicated by the differential exposure to potentially violent patients by staff members of large stature and strength. While some data have suggested that staff height/weight, gender, and training level are associated with assaults, there is much confounding of these data by self-selection or designation of responsibility to certain groups (e.g., large, young males). As such, prevention efforts should be directed at organizational and work environment factors rather than staff-specific characteristics.

ORGANIZATIONAL AND WORK ENVIRONMENT CHARACTERISTICS

As stated above, often staff-related characteristics are confused with organizational and work environment characteristics. For example, the risk of violence in any healthcare organization varies across job titles with nursing personnel, in particular with nursing assistants, who experience the highest risk of assault. This variation can be explained by the differential exposure to the hazard, as well as by organizational and work environment factors that place one group of workers at either increased or reduced risk.

Similarly, staff skills in the prevention and management of disruptive behavior is sometimes described as a staff characteristic but should be more accurately described as a work organization characteristic, related to the type and quality of training provided to staff. We believe that work environment characteristics, including job tasks and intensity of exposure to patients/clients, are more relevant to understanding why certain groups of staff are disproportionately victims of workplace violence.

Findorff, McGovern, Wall, Gerberich, & Alexander (2004) conducted a mailed survey of current and former employees of a major Midwest healthcare system. The 1,751 employees who completed the survey held a variety of jobs ranging from clinical positions to clerical and technical positions. The odds of physical violence were increased for patient care assistants (OR = 2.5) and nurses (OR = 3.8) and decreased for clerical workers (OR = 0.1) when compared with medical specialists that included physical and respiratory therapists and medical technicians. Adjusting for the amount of patient contact resulted in increased odds of physical and non-physical violence for patient care assistants, but not for nurses. Increased supervisor support decreased the odds of both physical (OR = 0.7) and non-physical violence (OR = 0.5), adjusting for job and demographic characteristics.

In a large survey conducted by the same research group, a sample of 6,300 randomly selected nurses in the state of Minnesota and a subsequent nested case-control study found annual rates of physical and non-physical assault (i.e., verbal) of 13.2 and 38.8 per 100 nurses, respectively. Cases were more likely than controls to report: higher levels of work stress; the belief that assault was an expected part of the job; witnessing all types of patient-perpetrated violence in the previous month; and taking corrective measures against work-related assault. The odds for assault were significantly increased in nursing homes and long-term care facilities (OR = 2.6), emergency departments (OR = 4.2), and psychiatric departments (OR = 2.0) compared with acute care hospital units. Risks were decreased when carrying cellular telephones or personal alarms (OR = 0.3). Controls were more likely to perceive higher levels of morale, respect and trust among personnel, and to believe that administrators took action against assaults (Nachreiner et al., 2007).

Welch, Hodgson, & Haberfelde (2012) reported on eight years of standardized assault incidence data among nursing staff working across VHA healthcare facilities. They found that female nursing assistants and licensed practical nurses experienced assaults at a rate 6.0 and 2.3 times higher risk than registered nurses.

RESTRAINT AND/OR SECLUSION IN BEHAVIORAL EMERGENCIES

The use of restraint and seclusion to protect both staff and patients from injury in the course of managing behavioral emergencies should be part of any discussion of violence prevention in health care. Professional organizations and certifying bodies have issued statements and recommendations expressing their commitment to the reduction and ultimate elimination of seclusion and restraint. Their position statements and standards, although based on the widely held principle of the ethical treatment of all individuals, in particular the most vulnerable among us, present a dilemma for staff who are held accountable for following such standards while managing behavioral emergencies in today's often under-staffed healthcare work environment.

It is well recognized that violence on inpatient units, particularly on psychiatric wards, often cannot be predicted and that in response to this reality, direct care staff, as well as RNs and other professional staff, often see seclusion and restraint as a necessary last-resort intervention to maintain that safety.

The 2014 APNA position statement on the use of restraint and seclusion states

> *Psychiatric-mental health nurses play a critical role in the provision of care to persons in psychiatric settings. This role requires that nurses provide effective treatment and milieu leadership to maximize the individual's ability to effectively manage potentially dangerous behaviors. To that end, we strive to assist the individual in minimizing the circumstances that give rise to seclusion and restraint use. (APNA, 2014)*

The statement goes on to articulate fundamental principles to guide action on the issue of seclusion and restraint.

Similarly, the American Nurses Association (ANA), in their 2012 Position Statement titled *Reduction of Patient Restraint and Seclusion in Healthcare Settings* states

To achieve a culture of non-use of restraints, facilities should adopt formal procedures and policies that clearly state the intent to promote a reduced restraint environment for patients. Such statements must include a focus on

1. *Intention to comply with policy standards;*

2. *Environmental designs to facilitate restraint reduction;*

3. *Sufficient registered nursing staff to monitor and intervene as needed; and*

4. *Implementation of an individualized approach grounded in the principles that a) all behavior has meaning, b) patient needs are best met when behavior is understood; and c) systematic approach of assessment, intervention, and evaluation is the best means to respond to behavior (ANA, 2012)*

The Statement concludes

There is a critical need to provide educational opportunities to assist nurses in developing the necessary assessment and intervention skills to reduce the use of restraint and seclusion. ANA is concerned that lack of personnel to provide adequate monitoring of patients and less restrictive approaches to behavior management may increase the violation of patients' rights and place them at greater risk of harm caused by being placed in seclusion and/or restraints. (ANA, 2012)

The Centers for Medicare and Medicaid Services (CMS) has published a rule (Code of Federal Regulations, 2006) and The Joint Commission a standard (TJC, 2009) requiring the evaluation and documentation of all patients' behavior-based restraint and seclusions.

In addition, a vast literature has examined the impact of restraints and seclusion on patient outcomes. One of the few studies to also address staff injuries found that the use of physical restraints was associated with injury to both patients and staff (LeBel & Goldstein, 2005). Our experience confirms this association.

We believe that it is critical to examine all of the factors that lead to the use of restraints and seclusions in a particular setting, both factors related to the individual patient, and organizational factors that may contribute to patient behaviors that then lead staff to consider the need to restrain or seclude patients.

STAFFING

Ensuring that there is adequate staffing is a critical work organization characteristic that must be part of any genuine strategy to prevent violence. Professional nursing, led by the ANA, has been actively involved in a national discourse, including research and health policy emphasizing the influences of staffing on the safety of both the patient and the nurse. There is also broad recognition that rising patient acuity and shortened hospital stays contribute to adverse patient and staff outcomes (see link to ANA's 2012 staffing principles in Appendix A).

A recent study and report by Yragui, Silverstein, Foley, Johnson, & Demsky (2012), conducted within two large Washington State Forensic Hospitals, is the first to examine workplace violence within the larger contexts of patient quality of care and worker quality of work. They found that low or inadequate staffing was related to many adverse outcomes, most relevantly to increased patient assaults, but also to worse health and work outcomes. Moreover, both measures of patient quality of care were linked to staffing adequacy, making it a critical organizational factor to target. Their qualitative findings support addressing staffing issues as well, and begin to clarify the complex dynamics of high disruptive behavior, low morale, increased and/or unscheduled absences, high turnover, and difficulty filling vacancies—all factors that reduce staffing adequacy and stability and increase risk of violence for patients and care providers alike.

In numerous focus groups we have conducted across four states, inadequate staffing is consistently identified as a major factor contributing to staff assaults. In addition, staff members describe fatigue from working overtime, especially mandatory overtime, and the impact of overtime on reduced ability to react with empathy and patience when clients are disruptive or their behavior is escalating. Staff also reported that inadequate staffing contributes to violence when staff members are not available emotionally for the clients.

Worker Rights and Legal Protections

WORKER RIGHTS AND LEGAL PROTECTIONS provided to workers vary by political jurisdiction, including by country, state, and sometimes even locally. Overall, particularly in the United States, owners and managers of companies (including healthcare organizations) continue to have a range of rights and prerogatives; this is true for private non-profit companies, like hospitals, and even for government agencies. Broadly speaking, these include the rights to

- Hire employees
- Direct, control, and assign work
- Establish schedules and hours of work
- Determine employee qualifications
- Establish and enforce rules of conduct
- Discipline and terminate employees for cause
- Expand and reduce the number of employees
- Lay off employees and recall from layoff
- Consolidate, transfer, or close operations/units

For the past hundred years, the power of owners and managers has been mitigated, at least somewhat, by a range of labor laws. Generally, those laws were enacted only after protracted political battles, generally waged by workers and unions.

The U.S. Department of Labor (DOL) is a cabinet-level federal U.S. agency with responsibility and authority for developing, promulgating, and enforcing most laws governing employee and employer rights and protections. The U.S. DOL lists nineteen categories of laws that they enforce. The first two are

- Wages & Hours
- Workplace Safety & Health

Wage and hour laws principally focus on ensuring that all workers are paid at least the minimum wage and that they are paid for the hours that they work, including overtime hours. These basic requirements are generally complied with by in-patient healthcare settings. For home health aides and hourly field-based workers, compliance may be more sporadic.

Regardless, where issues involving wage and hours intersect with safety and health is around the question of overtime. There is no federal regulation limiting the overtime that nurses can work. Some states, however, have enacted such regulations, principally for the purpose of safeguarding patient care. Those state-level regulations are typically enforced by the state's Department of Labor or Health. The rationale for these regulations is that healthcare workers' vigilance and performance is compromised when they are exhausted from working overtime, including back-to-back shifts for days on end. Not only is the risk of medical errors increased, but staff injuries can result when judgment is compromised. If a patient's behavior is beginning to escalate, the staff person may not notice the early warning signs of such behavior, may not have as much patience as they otherwise would, and may not be able to readily retrieve the information and de-escalation techniques taught during training.

Workplace safety and health regulations are principally the domain of the federal Occupational Safety and Health Administration (OSHA). OSHA is charged with adopting and enforcing workplace safety and health regulations. OSHA was legislatively created in 1970 under the Occupational Safety and Health Act (referred to as the OSHAct) following a series of high-profile workplace disasters with multiple fatalities, and by a protracted campaign by unions, environmentalists, and the public health community.

OSHA provides many protections, but there are numerous limitations, as well. It is important to understand both.

> **First—***Who* does OSHA cover? OSHA covers both for-profit and non-profit private employers in most employment sectors. A notable exception is people who are self-employed. Importantly, federal OSHA does not automatically cover public sector workplaces. Employees who work for state and local governments are not covered by federal OSHA, but may have OSHAct protections if they work in a state that has an OSHA-approved state program. Such a program must cover at least the same hazards as federal OSHA, and must be at least as effective. Only about half the states have such a state program and thus provide OSHA coverage for their public sector workers (see list of OSHA Plan States in Appendix C). Thus, if you work in a state without such a program, you will not be covered by OSHA if you work for a state agency, even if you are a healthcare worker within a state-run psychiatric hospital, facility for the developmentally disabled or public university-run medical center. Healthcare workers who work in federal facilities (e.g., VA hospitals) are covered under the Federal Agency Health and Safety Program.
>
> **Second—***What* does OSHA cover? The 1970 OSHAct begins with the phrase: "To assure safe and healthful working conditions for working men and women." It is the employer's responsibility to create such working conditions; however, OSHA does not require that employers have a comprehensive health and safety program that identifies and mitigates all workplace hazards. Instead, OSHA largely relies on hazard-specific standards or rules, such as the Blood Borne Pathogen Standard. Before OSHA can issue a standard, it must go through an extensive and lengthy process that includes substantial public engagement, notice and comment periods. This is known as OSHA's 'rulemaking process'. As a result, virtually no new standards have been enacted in the past twenty years. In fact, Congress has forbidden OSHA from taking action on many important hazards such as ergonomics, which includes safe patient handling. With regard to workplace violence, OSHA became interested in the issue in the 1990s and produced useful guidance documents, including "Guidelines for Preventing Workplace Violence for Healthcare and Social Service Workers" in 1996. However, OSHA has not initiated a rulemaking process for workplace violence prevention.

GENERAL DUTY CLAUSE

Section 5(a)(1) of the OSHAct, referred to as the "General Duty Clause," states that "Each employer shall furnish to each of his employees employment and a place of employment which are free from recognized hazards that are causing or are likely to cause death or serious physical harm to his employees. (OSHA, 1970)" OSHA can inspect, issue a citation, and fine an employer who does not comply with statement.

Several conditions must be met for OSHA to issue a General Duty Clause violation including:

- The hazard was recognized
- The employer failed to keep the workplace free of a hazard to which his or her employees were exposed
- A feasible and useful method was available to correct the hazard
- The hazard was causing or likely to cause death or serious injury

In practice, this means that for OSHA to issue a General Duty Clause citation for workplace violence, there must be an actual risk of workplace violence that has been observed; the work setting must be one where the risk of workplace violence is generally recognized (e.g. epidemiologic studies have documented the elevated risk within this type of setting); the risk must be serious; and there must be preventive measures that have been identified, and that the employer should have been aware of.

Until fairly recently, federal OSHA rarely used the General Duty Clause to inspect and cite hospitals for the hazard of workplace violence, in part because the political climate would not support such OSHA actions but additionally, because no guidance existed on how to conduct such an inspection. In 2012, OSHA took an important step toward beginning to address workplace violence in health care and other high-risk settings by publishing a compliance directive detailing the hazard in those settings and providing OSHA compliance officers with a guide to using the General Duty Clause to respond to complaints regarding the hazard of workplace violence.

Between 2011 and 2014, federal OSHA conducted 122 inspections in response to the hazard of workplace violence, 84 of which were in healthcare establishments (see Chapter 15).

PROTECTION FROM RETALIATION OR DISCRIMINATION

Section 11(c)(1) of the OSHAct is designed to protect workers from suffering discrimination or retaliation if they exercise their rights under OSHA. That section states

> *No person shall discharge or in any manner discriminate against any employee because such employee has filed any complaint or instituted or caused to be instituted any proceeding under or related to this Act or has testified or is about to testify in any such proceeding or because of the exercise by such employee on behalf of himself or others of any right afforded by this Act. (OSHA, 1970)*

Since there is a long history of retaliation toward workers that complain about working conditions, the compliance directive that accompanies New York State Workplace Violence Regulation addresses this issue as well. It states

> *The employer is also prohibited from taking retaliatory action against employees who exercise rights accorded by this rule. Retaliatory actions will be investigated as a PESH discrimination case. Note that retaliatory actions under this rule constitute a PESH act violation (NYS, 2009).*

Retaliation and discrimination do occur, and if you file an OSHA complaint and are subjected to such behavior, you should take the following precautions. Make sure that you document how you exercised your OSHA rights, what the retaliatory actions consisted of, obtain witnesses if possible, and obtain help from your union if you have one. Without a union, it can be quite challenging to defend yourself in these situations.

RIGHT TO COMPENSATION IF INJURED ON THE JOB

Another relevant legal right that workers have is the right to compensation if they are injured or made ill by their job. This is typically through their state's workers' compensation system. There is no federal workers' compensation system—instead each state has its own system and rules. Typically, this is insurance coverage that employers are required to carry.

Many times, a workers' compensation claim will be contested or controverted, either by the employer directly, or by his/her insurance carrier. The system is often complex, bureaucratic, and time-consuming. Once a claim is awarded, the worker's relevant medical costs will be covered, and they will receive at least partial compensation for lost wages. Temporary or permanent disability payments may also be awarded.

In most states, workers' compensation is the sole compensation remedy available to workers—they are barred from filing suit against their employer for unsafe working conditions.

In addition to these civil remedies, workers retain the right as an individual to seek criminal charges against those who commit a violent act, whether they are a patient, client, visitor, or fellow employee. Your employer should support and potentially assist you in such matters. They cannot prevent you from filing a police report. As discussed earlier, many employers may hold that "it's part of the job", or "the client didn't mean it." Unfortunately, many members of the criminal justice system may share that view, presenting obstacles in an injured worker's attempt to obtain justice. For this reason, if there is a serious persistent problem of workplace violence in your facility, it is important for the workers collectively, with their union and/or employer, to establish a productive working relationship with the local police, district attorney, and courts. Invite them to your facility. Get them to speak to some workers who have been assaulted. With enough education, they can usually be made to understand that assaulting a nurse is just as serious as assaulting a police officer or a judge—no assaults should be tolerated.

In the absence of a union, the National Labor Relations Act of 1935 gives employees the right to act together to try to improve their pay and working conditions, with or without a union. If employees are fired, suspended, or otherwise penalized for taking part in protected group activity, they can appeal to the National Labor Relations Board to restore these rights. Workers' rights to act collectively have been upheld in numerous decisions by appellate courts and by the U.S. Supreme Court (National Labor Relations Board, n.d.). However, these rights are much more easily utilized by and protected for workers who are in a union. Besides offering protection to workers who are treated adversely and unfairly by the employer, the union can negotiate with the employer about a range of working conditions, many of which are germane to workplace violence prevention. This can include: staffing, work rules, training, and the creation of a health and safety committee that includes union representatives and frontline workers, as well as managers.

Regulations, Laws and Voluntary Standards. How Can You Use Them to Your Advantage?

AS DESCRIBED EARLIER, there is no federal regulation or law addressing workplace violence and it is unlikely that there will be one anytime soon. In the absence of such regulations, we must look to states and voluntary certifying bodies (such as TJC) to provide leverage to advance worker protection.

STATE LAWS AND PROPOSED STANDARD

As of 2014, workplace violence laws addressing violence in health care and social assistance have been passed in a number of states (Table 1).

The most comprehensive U. S. workplace violence law is the one enacted in New York State (NYS). The law covers all public sector workplaces within the state, with the exception of K–12 schools, which are covered by separate Safe Schools legislation. The NYS law was passed in 2006, and the NYS DOL's final regulations, 12 NYCRR Part 800.6, were published in April 2009 and required compliance by August 27,

Table 1. Summary of U.S. States with Workplace Violence Laws

State	Date	Sector	Risk Assessment Required?	Employee Involvement Required?	Enforcement Agency
California[1]	1995, 2012	Hospitals	Yes	No	Health
Connecticut[2]	2011	Health care(>49 employees)	Yes	Some	Health
Illinois[3]	2008	MH and Dev Disability	Review Incidents	No	HHS & Health
Maine[4]	2012	Hospitals	Review Incidents	No	Not Specified
Maryland[5]	2014	Hospitals, Nursing Homes	Yes	Some	Not Specified
New Jersey[6]	2011	Hospitals, Nursing Homes	Yes	Yes	Health
New York[7]	2009	All Public except K–12	Yes	Yes	Labor
Oregon[8]	2007	Some Health care	Yes	No	Not Specified
Washington[9]	2000, 2001, 2007	Some Health care	Yes	No	Labor

[1] California Hospital Safety and Security Act (Assembly Bill 508)

[2] An Act Concerning Workplace Violence Prevention and Response in Healthcare Settings

[3] 405 ILCS 90 Healthcare Workplace Violence Prevention Act

[4] Sec 1.22 MRSA 1832

[5] Maryland House Bill 710, Senate Bill 483

[6] Violence Prevention in Healthcare Facilities Act, Assembly Bill 3027

[7] Workplace Violence Prevention Law: Section 27-b of State Labor Law

[8] Oregon Laws Chapter 397

[9] Workplace Prevention Law: Chapter 49.19

2009. The law draws heavily on the Federal OSHA Guidelines for Health Care and Social Services, originally published in 1996 and revised in 2004, directing employers to control workplace violence via a comprehensive programmatic approach. The key elements of a program should be management commitment and employee involvement; worksite analysis; hazard prevention and control; training and education; and recordkeeping and evaluation. Of note, the NYS law requires that the employer involve union representatives and/or other employees in key aspects of the development and implementation of the workplace violence prevention program. New York State (NYS) provides OSHA coverage to public sector workers through a state plan administered by the NYS DOL.

In 2014, CAL/OSHA, California's state plan agency, began work on a comprehensive workplace violence prevention standard that will cover all healthcare workers in the state of California. The standard is in response to Petition No. 538 (https://www.dir.ca.gov/oshsb/petition_538.html). This will be the first workplace standard (as opposed to a state law) to address the hazard of workplace violence. The standard will be enforced by CAL/OSHA.

VOLUNTARY CERTIFYING BODY STANDARDS

TJC, recognized as a major driver in care delivery in U.S. healthcare organizations, is a not-for-profit organization that accredits and certifies more than 20,000 U.S. healthcare organizations and programs. A healthcare organization's eligibility to received Medicare and Medicaid reimbursement depends on accreditation by TJC or alternatively the Commission on Accreditation of Rehabilitation Facilities (CARF). CARF accredits health and human services programs primarily in the areas of aging, behavioral health, substance abuse treatment, and child and youth services. Although widely viewed as a driver of quality in health care, TJC has come under criticism for their practice of notifying hospitals in advance of the timing of inspections, the fact that approximately 99% of inspected hospitals are accredited, and that their governing board has long been dominated by representatives of the industries it inspects. Both TJC and CARF historically have had a nearly singular focus on patient safety, without regard to worker safety.

In recent years, TJC has, however, issued several standards and statements relevant to protecting staff (as well as patients and visitors) from workplace violence. In 2010, they issued *Sentinel Event Alert 45: Preventing Violence in the Healthcare Setting*. This alert requires healthcare facilities to address the problem of violence and to develop a written plan describing how the institution provides for the security of patients, staff, and visitors alike. To this end, institutions are required to conduct risk assessments to determine the potential for violence, provide strategies for preventing instances of violence, and establish a response plan that is activated when an incident occurs (TJC, 2010). The 2010 Alert reported that since 1995, TJC's Sentinel Event Database included 256 reports in the category of assault, rape, and homicide (combined) and that there was a significant increase in incidents reported between 2007 and 2009 with 26 incidents in 2007, 41 incidents in 2008, and 33 incidents in 2009. They identified the following potentially causal factors: problems in the areas of leadership, human resources, assessment, communication, physical environment and care planning. The Alert included 13 suggested actions (see Appendix D).

In addition, TJC has other initiatives and/or statements that can potentially be used as tools for advancing the protection of healthcare workers from work-related violence. Their *Framework for Conducting a Root Cause Analysis and Action Plan* states "A root cause is typically a finding related to a process or system that has a potential for redesign to reduce risk" (TJC, 2013). Critically important to the process of conducting an analysis is the action plan. Each finding that is identified as a root cause should then be considered for an action and addressed in the action plan.

Many organizations advise healthcare organizations to support the use of root cause analysis (RCA) as a structured method used to analyze serious (patient-related) adverse events. Interestingly, RCA was initially developed to analyze industrial accidents, yet while RCA is now widely deployed as an error analysis tool in health care, it is primarily used to prevent future patient-related adverse outcomes, rather than events that cause worker injury. According to the Agency for Healthcare Research and Quality (AHRQ), a central tenet of RCA is to identify underlying problems that increase the likelihood of errors while avoiding the trap of focusing on mistakes by individuals (AHRQ, 2012).

The goal of RCA is thus to identify both active errors (errors occurring at the point of interface between humans and a complex system) and latent errors (the hidden problems within healthcare systems that contribute to adverse events). As such, RCA could be an important tool in preventing violence-related staff injuries.

Workers should be familiar with these approaches and collectively ensure that their facility's management or safety and health committee use these tools to facilitate a comprehensive risk assessment following incidents of violence.

Workplace Violence Prevention Program (WVPP): OSHA Guidelines

OCCUPATIONAL HEALTH AND SAFETY PROFESSIONALS address a multitude of potential workplace hazards on a daily basis. The risk varies by the workplace and type of work being performed. The hazards may include chemicals, dusts, lifting, slips and trips, falls, dangerous machines, extreme temperatures. Many healthcare workers are exposed to a number of these hazards. Hopefully your employer has effective programs to eliminate or mitigate those hazards. Workplace violence is a hazard that has similarities to many of those other hazards, but significant differences as well.

The main difference is that the hazard is another human being. Many employers use this undeniable fact to assert that the problem of workplace violence has always existed, and always will exist. They may further assert that this means nothing can be done to prevent it. We reject this assertion.

We base this on the belief that there are some essential similarities between workplace violence and other workplace hazards. Through concerted effort, there is much that can be learned about the hazard, e.g., who, what, where, when, and why, and that knowledge can be used to develop effective prevention measures. This requires a comprehensive approach and the development of a multi-faceted prevention program. It is this approach that is the core of OSHA's "Guidelines for Preventing Workplace Violence for Healthcare and Social Service Workers" published in 1996, republished in 2004, and undergoing revision in 2014.

So what do we mean by a comprehensive workplace violence prevention program (WVPP) and what form should such a program take? Essentially we're referring to a program that identifies risk factors for workplace violence faced by staff of a healthcare facility and then modifies the work environment to minimize these risks. No factor should be ignored, even if some would assert that the factor is inevitable (e.g., human nature), or unable to be changed (e.g., inadequate staffing). Even if not all factors can be fully remediated, they should at least be acknowledged and addressed to the extent feasible.

A comprehensive WVPP should include a written document that is reviewed and updated at least annually. However, that document should be based on a dynamic program that is adapted to respond to changing workplace conditions, serious incidents, and an ever-changing patient population. To be effective, the program should include input from all areas of the organization, all of which should have some ownership.

The program must have as its foundation strong management commitment and worker involvement. These foundational elements then support the other program elements, namely, worksite analysis, effective control of hazards, training, recordkeeping, and regular program evaluation. Worker involvement is important in any comprehensive illness and injury prevention program, but particularly in developing a WVPP. Frontline healthcare workers are skilled in recognizing patients who may be at risk of violence. Additionally, those workers are key in identifying prevention strategies that are effective, and that do not have unintended negative consequences, either to staff or patient safety or to patient care. In the following chapters we will discuss each of the elements in greater detail and provide examples and tools to help you develop the various elements that make up a comprehensive effective program in your organization. What follows is a brief description of the core elements.

Management Commitment and Employee Involvement—
Management commitment must be evident in the form of high-level management involvement and support for a written workplace violence prevention policy and its implementation. Meaningful employee involvement in policy development, risk assessment, joint management–worker violence prevention committees, post-assault counseling and critical incidence debriefing, and follow-up are all important program components. This should include front-line workers and, where a union exists, union representatives. Without both management commitment and employee involvement, it is unlikely that an effective program will exist.

Worksite Analysis—A worksite analysis is the foundation on which an effective program exists. This analysis should utilize all available data sources and be repeated, at least in part, on a periodic basis. Data sources include: OSHA logs, first reports of injuries, other incident reports, and workers' compensation data. This information can be invaluable in identifying trends and risk factors. These data are often supplemented by staff surveys and focus groups. Regular walk-through surveys of all areas of the facility should be conducted, and should include staff from each area and from all shifts. Special attention should be paid to those areas where assaults have occurred. A Safety Committee has an important role in assuring a robust worksite analysis. Such a committee should review and track incidents by organizational, environmental, patient, unit, and staff level factors. A Safety Committee or a Violence Prevention Committee is an ideal forum for direct care workers and managers to review and analyze incidents and to identify and evaluate prevention strategies.

Hazard Prevention and Control—Hazard prevention and control measures should be designed based on the risk factors identified above. The classic industrial hygiene hierarchy of controls should be followed (discussed in Chapter 10). To the extent possible, exposure to the potential violence should be eliminated. An example of this is transferring an unstable, violent patient to a different facility, one that is better equipped to provide care to such a high-risk patient. The next priorities for prevention are engineering and administrative controls. Engineering controls to be considered include: modifying the layout of admissions areas, nurses' stations, medication rooms, lounges, patient rooms, or offices; limiting access to certain areas; and evaluating all furnishings to ensure that they are not used as weapons. Administrative controls include: developing and implementing appropriate policies and procedures; code procedures; appropriate staffing levels; and providing regular training. Finally, personal protective devices may be warranted, such as issuing cell phones and personal alarm devices to workers.

Staff involvement is just as important in designing effective controls as it is in conducting a thorough worksite analysis. Front-line staff can help identify unintended consequences of various prevention measures, and can provide feedback as to whether implemented changes have been effective. Additionally, programs need to be in place to provide support to assault victims and to their co-workers.

These can include easy access to medical and mental health services, assistance with the workers' compensation system, and support in accessing the criminal justice system, when appropriate.

Training and Education—At the time of hiring and periodically thereafter, worksite- and job-specific training should be provided covering the risk factors, prevention measures, and relevant policies and procedures. This should be specific to the type of setting, rather than a one-size fits all training. For direct care staff, training should include skills in the early identification and management of aggressive behavior. Violence prevention training should also include information on the prevalence of violence in the healthcare and social assistance work setting, risk factors for staff assault, a description of the facility's written violence prevention program, how to report incidents, and participation in committees addressing patient-on-staff violence.

Recordkeeping and Program Evaluation—Recordkeeping and program evaluation are inextricably linked and should not only focus on incidents of physical and verbal assaults but also on near-misses. Reporting should be something that staff are actively encouraged to do. Reports should be followed up and investigated promptly, with the results reported to the individual who made the report. Obviously, employees should not be retaliated against for filling out an incident report or filing a workers' compensation claim. The reporting and investigation of incidents is a critical means of evaluating the effectiveness of the WVPP and of identifying control measures which need to be modified or implemented. Staff should be encouraged to report all incidents, regardless of their severity. The reporting and review of incidents should be a critical aspect of the risk assessment and hazard control process. The number and severity of incidents should be tracked to evaluate the impact of organizational, unit, and staff-level changes such as enhanced security procedures, renovations to units, as well as changes in the patient population. The facility's health and safety committee or workplace violence prevention committee should undertake a comprehensive program evaluation at least annually.

OSHA is currently in the process of updating their 1996 guidelines (anticipated publication in 2015) to reflect the variations that exist in different types of settings, and to ensure the guidelines incorporate newer, more effective ways to reduce the risk of violence in the workplace. OSHA is increasingly aware of the fact that the workplace setting determines not only the types of hazards that exist, but also the measures that will be available and appropriate to reduce or eliminate workplace violence hazards. The updated document will provide specific guidance regarding five types of settings:

- Hospital settings, including large institutional medical facilities;
- Residential treatment settings, including institutional facilities such as nursing homes, and other long-term care facilities;
- Non-residential treatment/service settings, including small neighborhood clinics and mental health centers;
- Community care settings, including community-based residential facilities and group homes; and
- Field work settings, including home healthcare workers or social workers who make home visits

The updated guidelines will continue to emphasize the importance of a written program for workplace violence prevention that has as its foundation the five elements described above and further detailed in subsequent chapters of this book.

Management Commitment and Employee Involvement

AS DISCUSSED EARLIER, managers have extensive legal rights with regard to the organization and workplace, and thus also have significant responsibility for workplace conditions. Additionally, as leaders of the organization, managers play an enormous role in establishing the organization's priorities, and in setting the overall tone. Just as importantly, managers have great, if not total, authority for the allocation of resources, deployment of staff, capital expenditures, and the development of policies. Thus, it only stands to reason that without full management commitment to workplace violence prevention, it would be almost impossible to have an effective program.

The importance of employee involvement may be less obvious, but it is just as critical to effective workplace violence prevention. Direct care workers and their representatives, through their accumulated experience, are critical to identifying high-risk patients, activities, work locations, times of day, and other factors. Merely reviewing injury and incidence logs, while important, can never provide the complete picture in the way that directly talking to frontline workers can. Additionally, preventive measures, such as changes to policies or procedures, to the physical work environment, or even to staffing may result in unintended consequences. As frontline workers, staff are in the best position to predict those adverse impacts, or at least to identify them rapidly once the intervention is implemented.

So what should management commitment look like? A high-level manager should spearhead the development of the workplace violence prevention policy and program. Even if they are not the top leader of the organization, they should still have the authority to act, and should have the ability to communicate directly with the top leader. Additionally, they should be given the personnel and fiscal resources necessary to discharge this responsibility. Assigning a low-level manager with little authority, interest, or experience in health and safety or violence prevention is a clear sign that the organization is not serious about this issue.

Meanwhile, employee involvement is just as critical. If a union is in place, the union representative, e.g., the local president or the health and safety chairperson, should work hand-in-hand with the management leader. Hopefully, workplace violence prevention is an issue that both managers and workers can fully agree on. If there is no union, a senior well-respected nurse or other frontline caregiver should fulfill that role.

Ideally, a standing workplace violence prevention committee will be formed, and the committee will be jointly chaired by management and the workers. Additionally, the committee should include both department heads and direct care workers from either all work areas, or from a representative cross-section. The workers should be from a variety of job titles, and hopefully from all work shifts. The committee, with full worker involvement, should participate in all aspects of the WVPP, including policy development, risk assessment, identification of prevention measures, development of training, development of programs for post-assault counseling, critical incidence debriefing, and also ongoing review and evaluation of the WVPP (See Appendix E for an example of work performed by joint labor and management workplace violence prevention committee).

Often management commitment to violence prevention is compromised by a healthcare organization's nearly singular focus on patient safety. This can be evident in a written workplace violence prevention policy and program that focuses on safety for patients and visitors to the exclusion of staff. Similarly, risks for employees may focus on worker-on-worker violence, rather than the risk of assault from patient or family.

The importance of management commitment as part of an effective WVPP has been validated by peer-reviewed research. In a large survey of 6,300 randomly selected nurses in the state of Minnesota and a subsequent nested case-control study, cases defined as nurses who had experienced a patient assault were more likely than controls to report higher levels of work stress and to report that assault was an expected part of the job. Conversely, nurses who had not experienced a patient assault were more likely to perceive higher levels of morale, respect, and trust among personnel. They also reported that their administrators were more likely to take action against assaults (Nachreiner et al., 2007).

In our work, we have found that program success has depended on the ongoing work of a dedicated group of individuals representing management, labor, and direct care workers whose focus has been on workplace violence prevention. These facility-level committees were responsible for developing, implementing and sustaining the effort within their facility.

Numerous specific indicators of management commitment and employee involvement in the violence prevention process were identified in our NYS work:

- Regular participation of senior leadership in ongoing workplace violence prevention project advisory groups and in Safe and Therapeutic Environment Program (STEP) meetings. The presence of upper management at these meetings validated the importance of the process, but also provided a direct and timely link between the committee and other agency and facility decision-makers. As a result, staff felt they had the commitment of upper management on the issue of violence prevention

- Presence of senior staff at all Preventing and Managing Crisis Situation (PMCS) training also signified the commitment of upper management and the commitment of the organization to violence prevention. One facility indicated that management not only attends PMCS to make introductory remarks but is also required to attend annual training as well

- The organization's strategic plan included violence prevention goals and initiatives of the STEP committee. This action impressed the STEP committee because the strategic plan is the blueprint for the future. The plan is less vulnerable to changes in staff and management and is a communication tool with consumers and state level administrators. The STEP committee viewed this action as a concrete indicator of management's commitment to on-going violence prevention activity

- Daily participation by upper level administrators in ward rounds and morning reports was seen as further evidence of management's day-to-day commitment to working with staff to understand risk factors and promote timely policies to prevent violence on the wards

- Management analyzed facility and agency violence-related incident and injury data. These analyses were then shared and discussed with staff and committee members. All agreed that open sharing of data promoted the team approach to reducing violence, resulting in a more trusting environment for discussion. Additionally, this enabled the committee to identify risk factors and trends, and allowed for robust discussions about a range of prevention measures

- Management worked with the staff and unions to educate the local police, district attorney, and judges about the reality of workplace violence. This included supporting staff who chose to press charges against individual patients who committed serious assaults against staff or other patients. These actions provided concrete evidence to staff that management cared about their safety, and motivated staff to report hazardous conditions and assaults

- Committee process and activities had slowly resulted in a culture shift toward greater trust. The committees provided a venue for management to demonstrate their responsiveness to workers' concerns and for enhanced employee involvement as a result of believing that concerns would be heard

- Allocation of resources for the whole workplace violence prevention process, including staff, training programs, modifications to the physical environment, is yet another indicator of management commitment

Genuine employee involvement is closely related to and as challenging to achieve and maintain as management commitment. Each influences the other, with employee involvement a strong indicator of management commitment. Additional evidence of employee involvement included:

- The ability of frontline workers from various disciplines and wards/departments to participate in the process was facilitated by scheduling meetings in advance and directing supervisors to free up all committee members from their regular responsibilities so that they could fully participate

- Regular communication via the committee process, the rounds process, and shift-to-shift communication to identify hazards and suggest control strategies

- Employees and management crafted improved procedures for medicating patients over objections, though often requiring a court order

- Finally, in many facilities a robust, compassionate program for post-assault response and support was created. Those who implemented such programs found that it improved reporting of dangerous situations and assaults, improved return to work of injured staff, and contributed to the overall WVPP

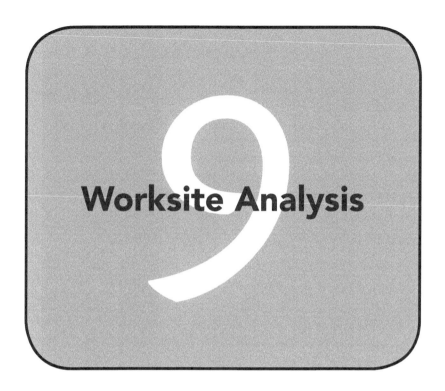

Worksite Analysis

A THOROUGH WORKSITE ANALYSIS is the foundation on which the subsequent program elements are built. It should combine basic industrial hygiene tools, e.g., a thorough review of the worksite itself, as well as how the work is actually performed, with a basic epidemiologic approach, investigating the incidents individually and collectively to learn Who? What? Where? When? Why? How? This analysis should be repeated on a periodic, or at least annual, basis.

The assessment can start with a review of available data, including OSHA injury and illness logs, first reports of injuries, other incident reports, and workers' compensation data. No single data source is likely to collect all relevant incidents. Collectively, the information can be invaluable in identifying trends and risk factors.

There is utility in designing a workplace violence incident reporting form that attempts to collect, in one place, much of the important information.

The NYS Workplace Violence Prevention Law mandates that the employer have such a form. The form must include, as a minimum

1. Workplace location where incident occurred
2. Time of day/shift when incident occurred
3. A detailed description of the incident, including events leading up to the incident and how the incident ended
4. Names and job titles of involved employees
5. Name or other identifier of other individual(s) involved
6. Nature and extent of injuries arising from the incident
7. Names of witnesses

This will facilitate the identification of trends and risk factors, such as high-risk work locations, tasks, time of day.

Often, and especially in institutional or long-term care settings, there may be a small subset of clients/patients that commit a disproportionate share of staff assaults. In one long-term care facility for severely developmentally disabled individuals where we provided consultation, we learned about a single client who had injured fifteen staff in the prior month. It is essential to closely monitor and track these incidents and focus control strategies on this group of clients.

It is also worth supplementing the data by conducting staff surveys and focus groups. These can provide rich information about the incidents themselves, about the need or effectiveness of post-incident support and reporting efforts, and of the effectiveness of existing prevention measures. Relevant clinical factors, including the diagnoses and treatment plans for patients that commit the assaults should also be considered.

A comprehensive workplace violence prevention program should include regular walkthrough surveys of all areas of the facility as part of an ongoing risk assessment, focusing on objects or conditions that could contribute to incidents of workplace violence towards staff. Ideally, direct care staff from each area and shift should take part in the survey or at a minimum, provide input into areas of concern or in need of assessment. Regular environmental walkthrough surveys of buildings, grounds and transport vehicles by facility maintenance staff and direct care workers will identify environmental risks for both client and staff injury. The walkthrough environmental survey should identify design, structural, mechanical, acoustical, and functional areas in need of improvement. Such a survey will allow the identification of items such as the availability of objects that could be used as weapons (i.e. glass display cases) that, if identified and removed, would materially reduce the hazard. Importantly, special attention should be paid to those areas where assaults have previously occurred (McPhaul et al., 2008).

The entire Safety Committee or Violence Prevention Committee should be involved in reviewing all of the above data and making decisions about prevention strategies based on the findings.

The approach taken by one NYS psychiatric hospital may provide ideas on how your facility can use data for prevention. They start by having an easy to use online form for recording all assaults, threats, and near-misses. They also track all uses of restraint and seclusion. For each incident, data regarding the circumstances surrounding the event are collected. The data are used on an on-going basis to inform clinical and organizational decisions, particularly data pertaining to serious incidents. Also, the aggregated data are analyzed and charted quarterly. Quarterly data for the last few years are included in the charts, graphs, and tables that are produced, and then provided to the entire committee for review and discussion. The data serve as both a risk assessment tool, but also as one way of measuring the effectiveness of the existing program. This can include identifying potential changes to the work environment, programming, policies and procedures, and even staffing. Obviously, this should also impact the content of the training that is provided, as well.

Examples of successful hazard assessment activities are as follows:

- Staff focus groups and/or staff surveys not only provide data on experiences with violence but often lead to engagement of staff in the process of preventing workplace violence, as well as improving communication between frontline staff and management
- Environmental audit reports have been used to develop and prioritize short- and long-term enhancements in the facilities. For example, environmental audit recommendations such as the need for communication devices (i.e., a drop phone in the nurses' medication station) and the need to secure furniture have received immediate attention. Changes requiring capital improvements have been evaluated in light of construction and renovation plans specific to each facility. Furthermore, the result was increased attention to the environmental factors during the violent incident de-briefing process

- Involving direct care staff (including technicians and aides) in the development and evaluation of clinical treatment plans not only improves communication about potentially violence patients, but also improves the quality and consistent application of the plan. It is generally agreed that patient care is improved when input from the direct care staff is a formal part of the care planning process

- Data collection and review are key to violence prevention programming. Where possible, there should be a system where incident and injury reports can easily be entered into a database. It should be expected that when organizations encourage and support the reporting of incidents they are likely to see an initial spike in the reporting of incidents. This should be seen as a success, rather than an indication that the problem is worsening

- Analysis of injury data in one facility led to an understanding of higher incidence of violence during evening shifts, in the dining room, and while patients were standing in lines. This institution changed its medication administration procedures to avoid patients waiting in lines. Other facilities have used the data to identify a small group of patients who were responsible for a large amount of staff injuries, injuries to other patients, and damage to the environment. This phenomenon of a few multi-assaultive patients being responsible for a disproportionate share of the facility's assaults is quite common

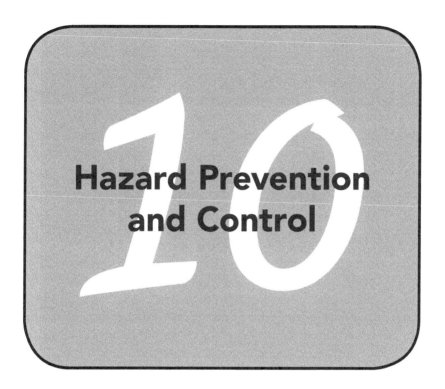

Hazard Prevention and Control

ENVIRONMENTAL AND WORK ORGANIZATION FACTORS are most amenable to modification and therefore should be a primary focus of hazard prevention and control efforts. A lack of security in high-risk areas, the presence of weapons in EDs, unsecured furnishing that can be used as weapons, hallways and patient care areas which have blind spots or do not allow passive surveillance, and poor lighting in outdoor areas are a partial list of such factors. Work organization factors that contribute to an environment in which violence can flourish include inadequate staffing, long patient waiting times, poor safety culture and a lack of staff empowerment and shared governance.

Unfortunately, there is no simple and universally effective way to prevent all workplace violence. The causes are complex; they vary by type of setting, type of patients/clients, and even from site-to-site and time-to-time. Certain principles and approaches are universal though and, if applied wisely, will help reduce the risk of workplace violence within your setting.

One principle in designing hazard prevention and control measures is to utilize a "hierarchy of controls," an industrial hygiene approach used to eliminate or reduce a wide variety of workplace hazards. This approach prioritizes, to the extent feasible, eliminating the hazard. An example of eliminating the hazard in a healthcare setting would be to substitute a less hazardous chemical for one that is more hazardous, such as the substitution of glutaraldehyde for formaldehyde. An example of reducing the risk of exposure to bloodborne pathogens to the extent feasible would include replacing traditional syringes with needleless devices.

Where elimination of the hazard is unlikely, as is largely the case with workplace violence in some high risk settings, the next priorities for prevention are engineering and administrative controls. Again, using the bloodborne pathogens example, the use of retractable needles is a relevant example. For workplace violence prevention, engineering controls to be considered include: modifying the layout of admissions areas, nurses' stations, medication rooms, lounges, patient rooms, or offices; limiting access to certain areas; evaluating all furnishings to ensure that they are not used as weapons. Administrative controls is another important category of workplace violence prevention. These can include: developing and implementing appropriate policies, procedures, and work practices; improving staffing levels to ensure that staff do not have to work alone and that there are sufficient staff to provide quality patient care while working safely; and providing regular and appropriately focused workplace violence prevention training.

The least preferred type of control, according to the hierarchy, is personal protective equipment (PPE). These methods rely on the compliance of all individuals, and often put a burden on the individual worker that should really be born by the organization as a whole. Examples include gloves, which can fail or cause dermatitis and other skin problems, and respirators, which are very uncomfortable and can make communication difficult. Where a hazard cannot be fully eliminated or controlled through the measures described above, PPE may play a legitimate and important role. Examples of PPE for preventing and controlling assaults include the issuing of cell phones and/or personal alarm devices (PAD) to workers. Cell phones can be particularly useful for staff that work in the field. They should be used in conjunction with an administrative control, a system for knowing where staff are working, and when they are scheduled to complete their field visit/assignment. It is also important to ascertain that cell service is available where the staff will be traveling and working. For institutional settings, the use of a personal alarm system can be useful. When activated, the alarm should indicate whose alarm it is, and the location at the time of activation. Obviously, security guards, a supervisor, or some other designated individual will need to be monitoring the alarms so that an immediate response can be provided. Those systems need to be tested regularly, and staff need to keep their PAD with them at all times.

Staff involvement is just as important in designing effective controls as it is in conducting a thorough risk assessment. Front-line staff can help identify unintended consequences of various prevention measures, and can provide feedback as to whether implemented changes have been effective. Staff have much expertise around how to work with individual and groups of patients while reducing the risk of injury and, therefore, they should be consulted about feasible control strategies that might not be available off the shelf or considered by management.

In some of the organizations with which we've consulted, staff were involved in all aspects of workplace violence prevention through a joint labor/management advisory group. This group was responsible for developing and implementing their violence prevention program. The group took the lead in developing hazard control action plans to address risks identified via the environmental survey, focus groups and staff survey. They were responsible for working with individuals and units to implement and track progress on hazard control activities and their impact on patient and staff outcomes.

Several types of assistance should be included in a post-incident response. Trauma-crisis counseling (which may include employee assistance program) should be readily available to the victim and other impacted staff. In addition, a separate process of critical-incident debriefing should be scheduled to discuss the circumstances surrounding the incident and what control strategies are needed to prevent future similar incidents.

POST-INCIDENT DEBRIEFING

Additionally, other resources that need to be in place to provide support to assault victims and to their co-workers include easy access to medical and mental health services, assistance with the workers' compensation system, and support in accessing the criminal justice system, when appropriate.

Flannery & Walker (2008) evaluated 14 empirical studies of the Assaulted Staff Action Program (ASAP), a voluntary, system-wide, peer-help, crisis intervention program for staff victims of patient assaults and found a 25%–62% reduction in staff assaults associated with the programs. The post-incident debrief process will contribute to the root cause analysis, as it will inform corrective actions needed to prevent future staff injuries.

Staff have much expertise working directly with individual clients and groups of clients. This expertise should be tapped following any incident in order to improve working conditions and client care.

Many healthcare organizations provide confidential employee counseling services as part of their overall employee benefits package. These employee assistance programs (EAPs) are intended to help employees deal with personal problems that might adversely impact their job performance, health, and well-being. EAPs generally include short-term counseling and referral services for employees and their household members. Many organizations and workers view their EAP as a valuable resource for employees following a violent incident. In our experience we have found EAP programs to have only limited effectiveness in this area. Typically, they focus on the individual, providing strategies for coping with the emotional and psychological effects of a violent incident. They often do not have the skills to place the individual response in the context of the larger problem of workplace violence and therefore are of limited value. Additionally, some workers may view EAP with suspicion, as supervisors may also refer employees based upon unacceptable performance or conduct issues.

ENGINEERING CONTROLS

As noted above, engineering controls are a critical first step in the prevention and management of workplace violence in health care. Ideally, these factors would be considered from the time that a building or ward is renovated, or even in its initial design. In our work with healthcare and social assistance organizations across four states, we collaborated with an architect who specializes in building security, and we developed an environmental survey checklist that can be used in patient care units (Appendix F).

ADMINISTRATIVE CONTROLS

A well-done study of an administrative control to prevent workplace violence was conducted by the VHA system. Their electronic mechanism for flagging a file of a patient who has committed violence against a staff person within the past two years led to a 90% reduction in assaults by these high-risk patients. The patient flag allowed workers to benefit from others' experience with the patients and take measures such as security stand-by, search for weapons, or patient confinement to one area of the hospital (Drummond, Sparr, & Gordon, 1989).

Any time that care for a client is handed off, such as at shift change, a clear system for communicating patient behavior must be in place to assure staff are informed of a change in a client's behavior which could place them or others in the setting at risk of injury.

Facilities where assaults are common should have a crisis response team, accompanied by a clear code procedure. The facility's code procedures should include not just medical codes, but also codes that correspond to specific levels of threat or out-of-control patients. All staff must be trained on how and when to initiate a code. There are different philosophies as to how the crisis response team should be composed. Some facilities want one team that covers the entire facility, with team members available on each work shift. The strength of this approach is that the facility can be more selective as to who is part of the team, and the training of the team can be more intensive. The weakness is that the response team, by coming from the entire facility, may take a bit longer to arrive, and may not include staff who are familiar with the patient(s) who is escalating and who has prompted the calling of the code. An alternative approach is to have a team from each ward or unit. This can put a burden on the staffing of the unit, e.g., remaining patients on the unit may have minimal staff or may be temporarily left once a code is called. Also, this approach requires that teams on each ward or unit receive sufficient training. Regardless of which approach is utilized, it is clear that all team members must have proper training (see below), and that clear procedures and responsibilities are delineated for the team and its members.

As described earlier, having sufficient staff is a critical element in having a safe workplace. One approach to ensure that staffing is sufficient in all wards and units during all shifts is to establish a float pool of permanent care provider staff, using the float pool to increase staffing adequacy, increase schedule flexibility and address unscheduled absences. This will reduce the use of overtime, which will likely save the facility money, and also ensure that staff are well rested as they care for their patients.

PERSONAL PROTECTIVE EQUIPMENT (PPE)

PPE is an appropriate control measure when engineering and administrative controls are infeasible or at least insufficient. Personal alarm and/or cell phones are essential forms of PPE that should be available to all staff working in high-risk settings and to all workers who work in the community setting. A discussion of the technical features of such devices is beyond the scope of this book. Critical features of the use of such devices as an effective hazard control include: a written procedure for how to access the personal device, plan for maintenance of devices, and how to obtain a replacement device when needed. We have found much variation in policies regarding the use of cell phones on the job. Many employers discourage or prohibit the use of cell phone on the job out of a concern that staff will use them for personal purposes while on the clock yet expect staff to use them to summon emergency assistance while transporting clients in the community. A written policy and the associated practice must include complete clarity on this issue.

Another form of PPE that may be appropriate when caring for individuals with developmental and mental disabilities are the use of gloves, sleeves, and blocking mats as a barrier method to protect staff from bites and scratches when other types of controls are infeasible. These types of protection are designed to reduce the possibility or severity of injury in the event of a client attack. Where the use of such protections are deemed necessary, the devices should be made of materials of high quality and must be well maintained and available to all staff on all shifts and at all times.

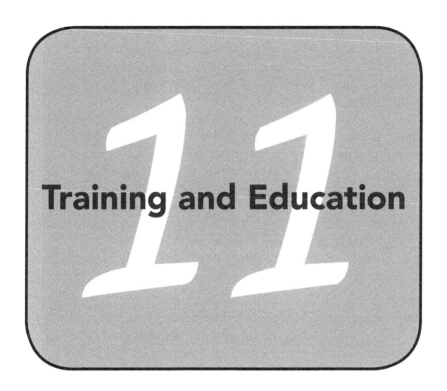

Training and Education

WHILE MANY HEALTHCARE INSTITUTIONS offer some workplace violence-related training, many of them, unfortunately, rely on this training as their primary or sole strategy for violence prevention. Although training is a necessary element of a comprehensive approach to address workplace violence, it is not sufficient on its own. More than 20 commercial workplace violence training curricula/systems are available from a range of vendors, and many large organizations have developed training curricula. Most of them focus on de-escalation and self-defense, with physical intervention techniques as a last report.

Effective workplace violence prevention training draws on the facility's complete workplace violence prevention program. It should be offered at the time of hiring and periodically thereafter, at least annually. It should be organization-, worksite-, and job-specific, covering the risk factors, prevention measures, and relevant policies and procedures for each worker. This should not be a generic training.

For direct care staff, training should include skills in aggressive behavior identification and management. Violence prevention training should also include information on the prevalence of violence in the work setting, risk factors for staff assault, a description of the facility's written violence prevention program, how to report an incident, as well as near-misses, threats, and other workplace violence concerns. The training should utilize adult education methods, making it interactive, with opportunities for staff to ask questions and to discuss actual and potential workplace violence scenarios. The facility's workplace violence or safety committee should be involved in reviewing the content of and method of delivery for the training. The curriculum should be reviewed and updated annually in the context of staff injury data. As part of orientation, staff should receive training on the prevalence of violence in this setting, risk factors for staff assault, a description of the written violence prevention program, how to report incidents, and how to participate and give input to committees addressing client on staff violence.

Additionally, for direct care staff in high-risk settings, there should be refresher training (with hands-on practice) in the prevention and management of crisis situations offered at least quarterly. Training should include hands-on practice of approved physical intervention techniques. It should address techniques to prevent the most common causes and types of injury, including bites and hair pulling. To ensure that staff are able to correctly and safely use these techniques in a crisis situation, it is critical that they are practiced regularly. Muscle memory matters. There should be remedial training available when an employee does not demonstrate adequate skills, and training skills should be reviewed and supplemented as necessary following an incident.

The Irish National Health Service has developed a highly structured approach to personal safety skills. They recommend that training at all levels of prevention should be participant-centered and include learning outcomes that are informed by a thorough risk assessment about the patient population, the staff/provider population, and the physical and social environment in which the interaction between them takes place (McKenna, 2008). While evidence suggests that training may reduce risks to staff, improve their clinical effectiveness, and result in cost savings, research into which specific training content and processes ensure safe, effective, and acceptable practice is severely limited. In the absence of national (or international) guidance on evidence-based education, training at all levels of prevention should be participant centered and include learning outcomes that are informed by a thorough risk assessment about the patient population, the staff/provider population, and the physical and social environment in which the interaction between them takes place.

In 2013, NIOSH developed and made available free of charge on their website a four-hour workplace violence curriculum targeting nurses (http://www.cdc.gov/niosh/topics/violence/training_nurses.html). The training was developed with broad input from numerous stakeholders, including the ANA and the authors of this book. According to NIOSH, the purpose of this course is to help healthcare workers better understand the scope and nature of violence in the healthcare workplace. Participants will learn how to recognize the key elements of a comprehensive workplace violence prevention program, how organizational systems impact workplace violence, how to apply individual strategies, and how to develop skills for preventing and responding to workplace violence. Content is derived from topic experts and from the OSHA 2004 Guidelines for Preventing Workplace Violence for Healthcare & Social Service Workers (OSHA 3148-01R 2004). The training has been well received and is currently one of the most frequently visited NIOSH web pages.

Federal OSHA has also recently engaged in a process of reviewing training curricula developed by nine vendors. The review is focused on the physical intervention techniques taught across curricula.

The following recommendations are based on our work across numerous populations and settings.

1. Curricula and training processes should include
    a. Clear definitions of what constitutes workplace violence and prohibited behaviors
    b. Review of the organization's workplace violence prevention program
    c. Where and how to report all incidents of workplace violence
    d. Theory and skills in the prevention and early intervention in potentially violent situations
    e. Self-protection techniques that may be performed by an individual staff member
    f. Physical intervention techniques requiring the presence of two or more staff
    g. Application and use of protective clothing and/or equipment

2. Curricula should be reviewed to identify the minimum number of staff needed to safely perform each intervention and training should explicitly state that the move should not be performed unless the minimum number of staff is available. Curricula should be reviewed to identify moves that can be safety performed by one individual and teach them as self-defense

3. Where possible, peer trainers should be used to deliver training

4. Training should attempt to incorporate real-life experiences to the extent that it is safe to do so. Where available, actual video of staff and patient interactions should be used in training and debriefings

5. All staff, all shifts, with patient care responsibility should be required to receive the training during work time

6. Procedures for summoning help in a behavioral emergency should be clearly defined, including who is leading the intervention (or code) and the role of security personnel

7. Training should be customized to special patient populations and settings. For example, community-based workers need specific training in how to remain safe when working in high-crime communities and/or making home visits. Some community-based workers have reported receiving very helpful training from law enforcement professionals

Recordkeeping and Program Evaluation

AN EFFECTIVE RECORDKEEPING PROGRAM is critically important, both in identifying risk factors and in determining what preventive measures should be adopted.

As described previously, the workplace violence incident report form can be in any format but, at a minimum, should contain the following information:

1. Workplace location where incident occurred
2. Time of day/shift when incident occurred
3. A detailed description of the incident, including events leading up to the incident and how the incident ended
4. Patient characteristics, including such information as diagnosis, history of violent behavior, violence triggers (if known)
5. Names and job titles of involved employees
6. Name or other identifier of any other individuals involved
7. Nature and extent of injuries arising from the incident
8. Names of witnesses

The form should be used to capture not only incidents of physical assaults and verbal threats, but also near-misses. Additionally, staff should have a mechanism for reporting workplace violence concerns, e.g., unaddressed risks that they identify. Reporting should be something that staff are actively encouraged to do. Reports should be followed up and investigated promptly, with the results reported to the individual who made the report.

Complete reporting and prompt investigation of incidents are critical means of evaluating the effectiveness of the WVPP and of identifying control measures which need to be modified or implemented. The number and severity of incidents should be tracked to evaluate the impact of organizational, unit, and staff-level changes such as enhanced security procedures, renovations to units, as well as changes in the patient population.

Facilities should compile and review their data quarterly, by facility, but also by other factors such as unit/location, time of day, staffing levels, and patient/perpetrator. In our experiencing, this recordkeeping has allowed facilities to evaluate and modify their program as needed. Specifically, it helps them understand where further interventions are needed as well as what control strategies are most effective, and to invest in those that have an impact on staff and patient injuries.

Working with Local Police and the District Attorney's Office

PARTICULARLY FOR FACILITIES that have frequent severe assaults that occur within the facility, it is important to develop a constructive relationship with the criminal justice system, particularly the local police precinct and department, and even with the local district attorney's (DA's) office (See Appendix G, Report from Norfolk, Massachusetts).

Unfortunately, too many police and DAs believe that if you work with "those people," you should expect to get assaulted. Those beliefs should be challenged directly. Nobody should expect to get assaulted at work. Certainly police, prosecutors, and judges would not stand for it if they were assaulted; they would ensure that the perpetrator was arrested, charged, and jailed. It should be emphasized that just because a person is mentally ill, developmentally disabled, or drunk, does not mean that they are incapable of making a conscious decision to threaten or assault. Therefore, they should be held accountable, just as other assailants are. Schenectady County (N.Y.) District Attorney Robert Carney said, "It's a common misconception, but patients can indeed have charges filed against them." He described a local case where a woman who worked for a Schenectady hospital's mental health services was stabbed in the chest with a pair of sewing scissors during a home visit, and his office successfully prosecuted and convicted her attacker (Commonwealth of Massachusetts, Norfolk District Attorney's Office, 2007).

One way to assist that educational process is to invite the members of the criminal justice system to your facility. Let them hear first-hand from direct care staff about what types of incidents occur. If possible, let them get onto the wards with staff to directly observe.

Communication should be ongoing between healthcare institutions and their local police departments as to what constitutes a crime, when the police should be called, who to call (specially appointed liaisons may be developed), and what happens when a crime is reported. It is critical that your organization provides: procedures for calling the police/activating the 911 system; procedures for filing criminal charges when assaulted and administrative assistance in filing criminal charges. Healthcare workers can report any crime, whenever and wherever it occurs. This is true whether the perpetrator is a patient, visitor, co-worker, or supervisor.

Healthcare institutions, including visiting nurse and hospice organizations, and law enforcement should work together to reduce workplace violence and to develop a plan in the unfortunate event that an emergency does occur. Meetings should be held to exchange contact information, basic knowledge of legal issues, and procedures for reporting threats or physical assaults. It may be preferable for healthcare institutions to designate one person as a liaison with law enforcement; similarly, local police departments and district attorney's offices should also designate a contact person for healthcare institutions.

A number of states and other jurisdiction have been successful in enacting legislation that makes violence against nurses a felony. Idaho recently passed such a law and violators could face up to three years in state prison if convicted. New York has a similar law, as well. Although such legislation draws attention to the problem of violence towards nurses (and other healthcare providers) we encourage nurses and their professional organizations to work toward more comprehensive legislation which focused on the prevention of violence in addition to consequences for offenders.

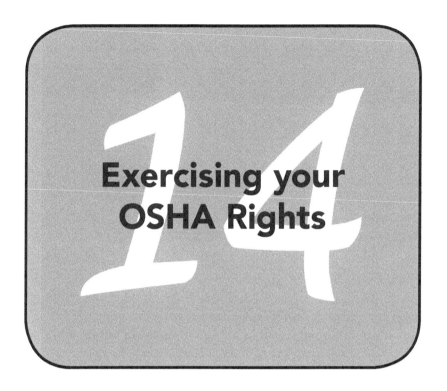

Exercising your OSHA Rights

IN CHAPTER 6, we discussed rights afforded workers by the OSHAct to protect them from workplace violence. In recent years, healthcare workers covered by federal OSHA have exercised their rights under OSHA's General Duty Clause to register a complaint and request an OSHA inspection for the hazard of workplace violence. In order for such a complaint to result in a successful inspection where violations are cited, the following criteria must be met: there must be an actual risk of workplace violence that has been observed; the work setting must be one where the risk of workplace violence is generally recognized, e.g., epidemiologic studies have documented the elevated risk within this type of setting; the risk must be of serious injury; and there must be measures that if implemented would reduce the risk of injury.

OSHA COMPLIANCE DIRECTIVE

In 2011, OSHA took an important step toward beginning to address workplace violence in healthcare and other high-risk settings by publishing a "compliance directive" detailing the hazard in those settings and providing OSHA compliance officers with a guide to using the General Duty Clause to respond to complaints regarding the hazard of workplace violence. An instance of workplace violence is presumed to be work-related if it results from an event occurring in the workplace.

According to OSHA:

> *This directive is not intended to require an OSHA response to every complaint or fatality of workplace violence or require that citations or notices be issued for every incident inspected or investigated. Instead, it provides general enforcement guidance to be applied in determining whether to make an initial response and/or cite an employer. (OSHA, 2011)*

The directive goes on to state:

> *Employers may be found in violation of the general duty clause if they fail to reduce or eliminate serious recognized hazards. Under this directive, inspectors should therefore gather evidence to demonstrate whether an employer recognized, either individually or through its industry, the existence of a potential workplace violence hazard affecting his or her employees. Furthermore, investigations should focus on the availability to employers of feasible means of preventing or minimizing such hazards. (OSHA, 2011)*

Between 2011 (partial year) and 2014 (through November 20, 2014), federal OSHA conducted 122 inspections in response to the hazard of workplace violence, 84 of which were in healthcare establishments. Among the 84 investigations in health care, 15 were issued 5(a)(1) citations, 38 were issued hazard alert letter, in 22 investigations there was no citation or letter, and in 9 cases the investigation is ongoing (cases can remain open for six months). OSHA may issue a hazard alert or letter to warn employers about the dangers of specific industry hazards and provide information on how to protect workers exposed to those safety and health hazards. Table 2 summarizes these 84 inspections by type of healthcare setting and outcome of investigation.

A sample of OSHA Press Releases summarizing the citations and settlement agreements issued over this period of time, summarized below, illustrate the type of violations that OSHA inspects/cites across a range

Table 2. OSHA General Duty Class Inspections and Citations (2011–2014*) (Total Number of WPV Inspections in Health Care Settings)

Year opened	2011	2012	2013	2014	Grand Total
5(a)(1) Citation	2	7	4	2	15
home	1	4	2		7
hospital			1	2	3
residential	1	3	1		5
Hazard Alert Letter	4	12	15	7	38
home	1		2		3
hospital	2	5	3	4	14
outpatient		1	1	1	3
residential	1	6	9	2	18
No citation or letter	0	6	13	3	22
home		1	1		2
hospital		3	5	1	9
residential		2	7	2	11
Ongoing investigation				9	9
hospital				5	5
residential				4	4
Grand Total	6	25	32	21	84

* 2011 (partial year), 2014 (through November 20, 2014)

of healthcare (Danbury, Armstrong) and social service agencies (Integra, North Suffolk).

Danbury Hospital in Danbury, CT, was cited by OSHA for failing to provide its employees with adequate safeguards against workplace violence. The OSHA inspection identified several instances during the past 18 months in which employees in the hospital's psychiatric ward, emergency ward, and general medical floors were injured by violent patients. OSHA found that the hospital's workplace violence program was incomplete and ineffective at preventing these incidents.

Armstrong County Memorial Hospital in Kittanning, PA, was cited with two violations following a complaint alleging that workers were suffering injuries from patient assaults in the hospital's behavioral health unit. One serious violation was for hazards associated with the employer's failure to implement programs and procedures to protect workers from injuries resulting from assaults by patients.

Integra Health Management of Owings Mills, MD, was cited for two violations following an incident when a service coordinator was fatally stabbed in Dade City by a patient in front of the patient's home. The employee was meeting the patient for a required face-to-face hospitalization risk assessment. The patient had a criminal history of violent behavior. A serious safety violation has been cited for exposing employees to incidents of violent behavior by a patient that resulted in death.

North Suffolk Mental Health Association Inc., in Boston, MA, was cited and entered into a companywide settlement agreement to implement comprehensive procedures and policies to better safeguard its workers against the hazards of workplace violence. OSHA cited North Suffolk for failing to provide adequate safeguards against workplace violence following the death of a worker in January 2011. A resident of the company's group home in Revere allegedly abducted and murdered the worker, who worked on-site as a senior counselor. (See Appendix G for a more detailed description of the citations).

Most of What We Know We Learned from Talking to Workers!

IN THE COURSE OF 15 YEARS of field work directed toward understanding and reducing the hazard of workplace violence in healthcare and social assistance workplaces, we have been privileged to meet with thousands of workers who have dedicated their careers (and often risked their lives) to care for individuals who suffer from mental illness, developmental disabilities, brain damage, other cognitive limitations, and/or substance abuse disorders. They strive to provide high-quality and compassionate care despite the difficult odds of doing so in light of serious cutbacks in funding at the federal, state, and local levels. In over fifty focus groups with workers across these settings we have heard heartbreaking and heroic stories of the challenges and successes these workers face on the job.

Interestingly, but perhaps not surprising, we found much agreement on the etiology of the unsafe working and patient care conditions across settings and staff. Common themes emerged from discussions with labor, management, consumers, and direct line staff across settings (in-patient, out-patient, and community), geography (rural vs. urban), and across experience levels and job titles.

We have attempted to summarize some of these recurring themes in this book. Although many of these refer to the mental health setting, we believe that they are relevant to all of healthcare and social service as patient/client acuity levels and caseloads increase as funding and other types of staff resources are reduced.

- A respectful and effective therapeutic relationship is the foundation for caring for the mentally ill. The ability to form and sustain therapeutic relationships is compromised by high caseloads, burdensome paperwork, and highly stressful work environments

- Caseloads have increased and many case managers believe that this increase diminishes the effectiveness of case management and other services by causing staff burnout, reduced ability to develop trusting and therapeutic relationships with patients, less knowledge of patient history, and pressure to cut corners or conduct home visits alone

- Clients who are more acutely ill often have co-occurring substance abuse disorders, and are much more likely to be violent

- It is difficult and sometimes impossible to obtain relevant information pertaining to a client's past history of aggression, assault, and criminal behavior. There is usually no time to search for this information in the files, and often databases are incomplete

- Staff safety training is critical, but many staff report receiving little or no safety training, inconsistent safety policies, or no regularity in training. In addition, the content of safety training is inconsistent across the system

- Knowledgeable and supportive supervisors and upper management are seen as extremely important to staff safety

- Conflicting philosophies of care often exist between clinical staff and direct care staff resulting in inconsistent boundaries and treatment of patients by staff and of staff by supervisors

- Poor and inadequate communication between treatment team members and direct care staff lead to inconsistent approaches to client behaviors

Special Case of Home Visiting by Community Health Workers

PROTECTING HOME VISITING MENTAL HEALTH WORKERS from violence while in the field presents substantive and complex challenges that must be recognized. First, each home entered by the worker is a unique and often unpredictable work environment. Unlike institutional settings, there are no security guards screening for weapons and contraband, there are no alarm systems or panic buttons, there are no video monitors, mirrors, special lights, quick release locks, drop phones or secure rooms, and no additional staff to attend to an agitated patient.

Home visiting pushes the limits of traditional safety programming practice. By contrast with the institutional setting where staff witness client behaviors on a 24-hour basis, home visitors obtain information by phone or other sources and conduct visits blind to the patient's immediate history, status, and behavior, and often past criminal history. Home visiting mental health workers routinely conduct visits without the benefit of either their own or their colleagues' professional assessment. Granted, the majority of mentally ill clients living at home do so because their condition is stable, but clients decompensate and may become high-risk to a home visiting worker. It is critical to have a system for identifying high-risk visits based on the research evidence, clinical recommendations, and community input, ensuring that those home visits are conducted by a pair of workers. Unfortunately, visiting in pairs is often not an option or not practiced in light of high caseloads and the shortage of staff available to work in pairs. As a result, a number of extremely experienced community mental health workers have lost their lives when visiting clients in their homes.

In 1998, a community mental health nurse, Judy Scanlon, was murdered by a client while visiting the client's home. This tragedy led to a number of activities, including much of the work described in this book. The murder was also the impetus for the New York State Workplace Violence law that we cited earlier this book. As required in the OSHAct, an occupational fatality triggers an investigation by the OSHA. In this case, the state OSHA-equivalent for public employees launched an investigation into this apparent occupational homicide. The nurse was a member of a union whose health and safety department provided substantial public pressure and leadership for both penalties for the employer and remediation to benefit all mental health field workers.

At the time, there was not a state law regulating violence hazards in the workplace. The employer, however, was cited by the state OSHA program for failure to provide a safe and healthful workplace under the difficult to enforce General Duty Clause. As noted earlier, in order for a citation under the General Duty Clause to prevail, there must be a hazard and the hazard must be recognized, there must be harm to employees, and there must be a means to abate the hazard. Therefore, it is significant that the employer was cited for workplace violence and that hazard abatement was considered recognized and feasible. The landmark case required the employer, a state mental health agency, to provide the following safety measures (remediation) for all of their visiting mental health workers employed throughout the state.

1. Regular training for dealing with potentially assaultive patients
2. An accountability system to track the whereabouts of all employees assigned to the field
3. Formal protocols to be followed by the visiting mental health nurses when conducting home visits which provide for their safety including adequate communication of such protocols to the employees

4. Accompanied visits when the patient's history indicates assaultive behavior
5. A means to summon assistance when necessary

Tragically, Judy Scanlon's murder was only the first of several workplace homicides that we would be asked to consult about. In 2002, Nicole Castro was murdered while visiting a client in Rockville, MD; in 2006, Marty Smith was murdered in Seattle, WA, again while visiting a client in the home. Fieldwork we conducted following Marty Smith's death elucidated the following risk factors for staff working in the community setting.

- **High caseloads (low staffing) and sicker clients**—Workers, patients, and managers alike agree that cutbacks and cost shifting in mental healthcare funding have resulted in higher caseloads and sicker clients. Budget cuts to mental health care mean more clients per worker. Furthermore, staff, consumers, and managers agree that reduced funding forces the system into prioritizing services for the acutely ill, leaving care for the chronically mentally ill and preventive and early intervention care largely unfunded. According to workers, higher caseloads translate directly into reduced time for case management and therapy for clients. Reduced time for each client means less time to read their history, if there is one, or search databases for information about a previous history of violence. Higher caseloads mean shorter, or less frequent, appointments, reducing the likelihood that the client will develop a trusting relationship with the caregiver. Shorter initial appointments are especially problematic. The first visit may be the client's first encounter in the community post hospitalization

- **Sicker clients**—Currently, services focus on the acutely ill rather than on the chronic needs of the mentally ill. This means that, in many cases, a person's mental illness has been allowed to progress without care until their condition is acute and life-threatening. Thus, patients are sicker by the time they receive care in the current system. Even community care clients are often dangerously ill by the time they are eligible for services. Furthermore, acute hospitalizations, according to staff, are not long enough to return the patient to baseline or to independent functioning in the community. Community supports are weak, resulting in clients who are not quite ready for the community but are discharged nonetheless

- **Paperwork burdens compete with client care**—Case workers unanimously feel that their high caseloads prohibit them from providing the kind of care they were trained to provide. Some former case workers report switching to other jobs within the system, such as crisis team worker, where they do not take a caseload but handle only emergency decisions for involuntary commitment. Workers reported that the stress and job dissatisfaction arising from increased caseloads, as well as the related paperwork burdens, have resulted in high turnover and high vacancy rates according to some staff. Qualified workers are changing jobs within the field, and some are even leaving mental healthcare altogether. Staff vacancies often result in an inexperienced, highly stressed workforce, and continue the vicious cycle

• **Management emphasis on productivity**—A related issue concerns staff perception that productivity rather than safety or quality is the primary concern of management. The reduction of services for early intervention and treatment is combined with higher caseloads for both inpatient and community mental health workers. The current reimbursement scheme emphasizes productivity in terms of actual patient encounters but does not account for missed visits, clients who are not at home, travel time, and clients who require more intensive time and effort

• **Incomplete access to client history of violence and criminal background**—In the aftermath of Marty Smith's tragic death, administrators at Kitsap Mental Services began to investigate the barriers to obtaining relevant information such as a client's past criminal history and evidence of past violent behavior. The problem is that some of this information goes beyond what is generally available in the clinical record, but may be relevant to both client and staff safety. In Marty Smith's case, relevant information about several past episodes of violent behavior involving law enforcement was not known to Mr. Smith when he decided to visit alone. This type of information is critical for all psychiatric care workers, but is of the utmost importance to community-based mental health workers. Substantive barriers to accessing this information continue to exist. Issues of confidentiality, civil liberties, and interagency cooperation (i.e., justice and social services) have been raised and will have to be systematically addressed in order to improve access to information so critical to worker and community safety

• **Mental health system deficiencies: Client access to medications**—Mental health workers lament that poor medication compliance is often a reason for decompensation and acute illness. Reasons for inadequate access to medications appear complex but related to cost, ease of access, eligibility for low cost drugs, entering the criminal justice system, and healthcare provider availability. Suffice it to say, that without appropriate medications, many mentally ill persons will suffer relapses of their disease resulting in behavioral symptoms (i.e., violent acts)

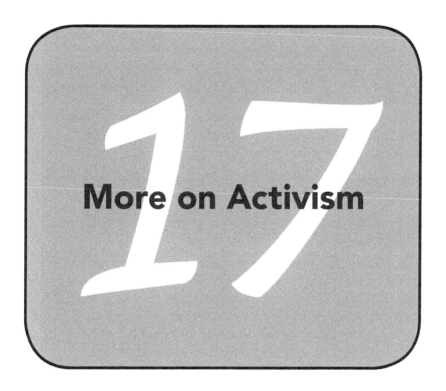

More on Activism

WE HOPE THAT BY THIS POINT IN THE BOOK, it is clear that a comprehensive and participatory approach to violence prevention in healthcare is essential to reduce workplace violence and provide the highest quality of patient care. The importance of including staff nurses and other front line workers in developing, implementing and evaluating a violence prevention program cannot be over estimated. We believe that nurses and other direct care workers need to come together collectively in their worksites to advocate for (actually, demand!) greater protections for themselves and by extension, their patients.

We urge RNs and other clinical staff to involve and work closely with direct care staff (e.g., health techs or aids) in all phases of violence prevention efforts. As you know better than most, patient behaviors may change from hour to hour and in response to various clinical, environmental and interpersonal factors. In many settings, direct care workers spend the greatest amount of time with patients, and therefore they are often in the best position to assess and evaluate behaviors and individual patient triggers. Their expertise is needed and therefore they should be actively recruited to serve on violence prevention and health and safety commit-tees. In addition, their involvement in such activity improves communi-cation among treatment team members and encourages the reporting of violent incidents or near-misses. Evidence suggest that when staff are provided the opportunity to use their expertise to impact programs, they perform at a higher level and are overall more satisfied with work. Patient care is also likely to improve.

ANA itself has excellent resources on its website to assist nurses in their advocacy:

http://www.nursingworld.org/MainMenuCategories/Policy-Advocacy/ State/Legislative-Agenda-Reports/State-WorkplaceViolence

We have also shared examples of such actions that professional nursing associations have taken to address workplace violence. We urge you to connect with the professional group that best represents your practice and get involved. Become a member if you are not already one; serve on a workgroup; run for office; testify before government bodies; write your elective officials; share your experiences with the public via editorials in your newspaper. But get involved.

Toward that end, we have also shared a number of such actions that we the authors have taken to draw attention to the issue and inform policy-makers regarding what needs to be done to protect nurses and patients from violence on the job (Testimony before a State Legislature—(see Appendix I and Appendix J, *Baltimore Sun* Op Ed).

Please consider this book a call to action.

Suggested Links and Resources

ANA Principles for Nurse Staffing, 2nd edition. (2012). A PDF of this is available free to ANA members. Others can order the publication at http://www.nursesbooks. org/Main-Menu/Specialties/Staffing-Workplace/eBook-Principles-Nurse-Staffing.aspx

American Psychiatric Nursing Association, , APNA Position on the Use of Seclusion and Restraint:
http://www.apna.org/i4a/pages/index.cfm?pageid=3728#sthash.T5eak2G6.dpuf

ASIS International, Healthcare Security Council issued "Managing Disruptive Behavior and Workplace Violence in Healthcare" in 2010. https://www. asisonline.org/Membership/Member-Center/Councils/hcs/Pages/default.aspx

ECRI Institute, an independent nonprofit organization that researches best practices to improve patient care, issued "Violence in Healthcare Facilities" in 2011 that discusses strategies for: preventing violent incidents; managing situations to prevent escalation; and enhancing the physical security of institutions. https:// www.ecri.org/Documents/RM/HRC_TOC/SafSec3.pdf

Emergency Nurses Association (ENA) Tool Kit:
http://www.ena.org/practice-research/practice/violencetoolkit/Documents/ toolkitpg1.htm

The Joint Commission article, Preventing Violence in the Health Care Setting: http://www.jointcommission.org/assets/1/18/SEA_45.PDF

National Institute for Occupational Safety and Health; Free Online training with continuing education CE (2013): www.cdc.gov/niosh/docs/2002-101/

Norfolk MA District Attorney William R. Keating Report on WV: The purpose of this document is to serve as a guide to help employers and law enforcement recognize the frequency and severity of workplace violence in healthcare, assess the risk of violence in the institutions they serve, and work together to develop workplace violence prevention programs and reporting mechanisms tailored to their institution's specific needs.

Occupational Safety and Health Administration: www.osha.gov/SLTC/workplaceviolence/

Link to guidelines: https://www.osha.gov/Publications/OSHA3148/osha3148.html

Link to compliance directive: https://www.osha.gov/OshDoc/Directive_pdf/CPL_02-01-052.pdf

Link to coverage for federal employees: https://www.osha.gov/OshDoc/data_General_Facts/federal-employee-factsheet.html

Washington State Department of Labor and Industry Workplace Violence Prevention: http://www.lni.wa.gov/Safety/Topics/AtoZ/WPV/default.asp

BULLYING RESOURCES

American Nurses Association on Violence and Bullying: http://www.nursingworld.org/FunctionalMenuCategories/MediaResources/PressReleases/2012-PR/ANA-Publication-Bullying-in-the-Workplace.pdf

International Association on Workplace Bullying & Harassment (IAWBH): http://www.iawbh.org

Washington State Department of Labor and Industry: http://www.lni.wa.gov/Safety/Research/Workplacebullying/Default.asp

Workplace Bullying Institute: http://www.workplacebullying.org

Workplace Bullying Bill: http://healthyworkplacebill.org/blog/tag/david-yamada/

APNA 2008 Report Recommendations

- The American Psychiatric Nurses Association released its position statement on workplace violence in October 2008. It included these seven recommendations applicable to workplace violence in all settings. Professional nursing organizations must advocate for (a) safe work environments, (b) education about risk management and prevention, (c) research support, as well as (d) stricter laws and mandatory regulations enforcing safe work practices

- Health organizations must establish and maintain a comprehensive program for the prevention, reporting, and management of all types of workplace violence

- Nurse managers need to create and maintain supportive work environments where respectful communication is the norm, organizational policies are followed, and incident reporting is efficient and blame-free

- Individual nurses should intervene when they witness aggression among their colleagues, recognize factors that may predispose patients to becoming violent, and report all incidents of violence

- Nursing educators must include workplace violence prevention and conflict management in the curriculum and prepare professional nurses in the prevention, assessment, and management of aggression in patients, visitors, and colleagues

- Investigators should study proactive prevention and intervention strategies, efficacy of training modalities, and efficacy of specific policies and leadership styles to identify best practices for prevention of workplace violence
- Researchers and clinicians must develop consistent and operationally defined definitions of what constitutes acts of violence in healthcare settings

States with OSHA State Plans

- Alaska
- Arizona
- California
- Connecticut
- Hawaii
- Illinois
- Indiana
- Iowa
- Kentucky
- Maryland
- Michigan
- Minnesota
- Nevada
- New Jersey

- New Mexico
- New York
- North Carolina
- Oregon
- Puerto Rico
- South Carolina
- Tennessee
- Utah
- Vermont
- Virgin Islands
- Virginia
- Washington
- Wyoming

NOTE: The Connecticut, Illinois, New Jersey, New York, and Virgin Islands State Plans cover state and local government workers only.

The Joint Commission's Suggested Actions

The following are suggested actions that healthcare organizations can take to prevent assault, rape and homicide in the health care setting. Some of these recommendations are detailed in the *HRC (Human Resource Control)* issue on "Violence in Healthcare Facilities" (TJC, 2010).

1. Work with the security department to audit your facility's risk of violence. Evaluate environmental and administrative controls throughout the campus, review records and statistics of crime rates in the area surrounding the health care facility, and survey employees on their perceptions of risk

2. Identify strengths and weaknesses and make improvements to the facility's violence-prevention program (The HRC issue on "Violence in Healthcare Facilities" includes a self-assessment questionnaire that can help with this)

3. Take extra security precautions in the Emergency Department, especially if the facility is in an area with a high crime rate or gang activity. These precautions can include posting uniformed security officers, and limiting or screening visitors (for example, wanding for weapons or conducting bag checks)

4. Work with the HR department to make sure it thoroughly prescreens job applicants, and establishes and follows procedures for conducting background checks of prospective employees and staff. For clinical staff, the HR department also verifies the clinician's record with appropriate boards of registration. If an organization has access to the National Practitioner Data Bank or the Healthcare Integrity and Protection Data Bank, check the clinician's information, which includes professional competence and conduct

5. Confirm that the HR department ensures that procedures for disciplining and firing employees minimize the chance of provoking a violent reaction

6. Require appropriate staff members to undergo training in responding to patients' family members who are agitated and potentially violent. Include education on procedures for notifying supervisors and security staff (4)

7. Ensure that procedures for responding to incidents of workplace violence (e.g., notifying department managers or security, activating codes) are in place and that employees receive instruction on these procedures

8. Encourage employees and other staff to report incidents of violent activity and any perceived threats of violence

9. Educate supervisors that all reports of suspicious behavior or threats by another employee must be treated seriously and thoroughly investigated. Train supervisors to recognize when an employee or patient may be experiencing behaviors related to domestic violence issues

10. Ensure that counseling programs for employees who become victims of workplace crime or violence are in place

Should an act of violence occur at your facility—whether assault, rape, homicide or a lesser offense—follow-up with appropriate response that includes:

1. Reporting the crime to appropriate law enforcement officers

2. Recommending counseling and other support to patients and visitors to your facility who were affected by the violent act

3. Reviewing the event and making changes to prevent future occurrences

State-Run Psychiatric Hospital Joint Labor–Management Committee (selected meeting minutes)

- Assaulted Staff Action Program (ASAP) – The frequency of patient-to-staff assaults continues at relatively lower levels than in previous years. As reported to ASAP, the majority of assaults in the past three months occurred on Unit G. In March 2012, ASAP counted 12 assaults with 5 on Unit H, 6 on Unit J, and 1 on Unit K. April saw 7 assaults (vs. 13 in 2011) with 4 on Unit H, 1 Unit J, 1 Unit M, and 1 CIU. So far in May, there were 5 reported assaults, 4 on Unit H, 1 on Unit J. We are down in ASAP volunteers for a number of reasons; I'll be recruiting volunteers across shifts

- Since many minor assaults occur on Unit H, the staff are tracking the frequency of these assaults and noted 15 incidents between 3-28-12 and 4-27-12 (vs. 32 in December 2011), with one patient (S) accounting for 8 incidents. Five other patients accounted for 7 incidents during this time. Our concern is the cumulative effect on staff who are most affected: one MHA was assaulted 5X, one RN day shift was punched in face, stomach, or spit at 4X. Another episode on April 27th involved a patient throwing feces and soiled towels at staff. Ideas from staff include specialized training in moving and positioning non-ambulatory patients especially for "float" staff who may not have been trained with addressing the needs of this population, as well as a more specialized training that would be dedicated to patients' needs and staff safety on this unit

- Staff X has compiled detailed comparisons between the frequency of assaults/ responses by ASAP with incident data found in the hospitals incident reporting system. He has detailed data for the past one to two years, with summary data for the past four years. ASAP records and responds to many more "incidents" than is noted in the system, which is as it should be. ASAP is concerned with staff's response and cumulative well-being regardless of degree of harm within a particular incident

Environmental Checklist: Violence Prevention Project

ARCHITECTURAL RESOURCES INC. BUFFALO, NY

Creating a Safe Environment: Ward Survey Checklist

1. Meet with faculty, staff and labor representatives
   a. Discuss concerns, incidents, resources and priorities
   b. Collect specific incident and injury data
   c. Identify a survey facilitator
   d. Combine the survey process with an examination of policies and procedures
   e. Schedule ward surveys and follow up process

2. Meet with individual ward staff
   a. Explain the goal of creating a safer work environment
   b. Review the process and schedule
   c. Discuss the layout of the ward and its ability to support the therapeutic program

d. Review ward specific incidents

e. Review ward specific conditions and construction details

f. Discuss daily routines and staff assignments

g. Review incident procedures

h. Describe a process for ongoing input and comments

3. Survey the ward

a. Entry area

i. Locking procedures and locking mechanisms

ii. Sally port?

1. Visibility

2. Duress communication

b. Circulation

i. Eliminate alcoves

ii. Visibility from control points

c. On-ward offices

i. Locking provisions

ii. Visibility

iii. Duress communication

d. Nursing stations

i. Discuss type and level of security/protections

ii. Maximize view and supervision

iii. Security for equipment and supplies

iv. Off-ward duress communication

v. Emergency medical/fire safety equipment

e. Program areas

i. Space and furniture configuration to support small groups

ii. Isolate noise generators (TV, stereo, active programs)

iii. Visibility

iv. Acoustics

Norfolk, MA District Attorney William R. Keating Report (excerpted) on Workplace Violence, 2007

CONTACT THE LOCAL POLICE—Crimes against the person should be reported to the local police department immediately. The police can assess the situation, gather evidence, take photographs and obtain statements from the victim and witnesses while everyone is still present and the incident is fresh in their minds. The police will determine if there is sufficient evidence to pursue criminal prosecution.

Healthcare workers may also go to the local police department after their shift to fill out a report or complaint. Reports or complaints must be filled out at the Police Department in the town where the incident took place.

Contact the Norfolk District Attorney's Office—There is always an on duty attorney or Massachusetts State Police trooper to answer questions or advise where to get answers. They can be reached at 781-830-4800.

Victim Witness Advocates—The vast majority of victims of a crime have no prior experience dealing with the criminal justice system. Victim Witness Advocates are trained professionals who help support victims and witnesses of a crime. Some of the services they provide include: Keeping victims/witnesses informed of the progress of the case; providing crisis intervention and emotional support; providing referrals for financial, medical, counseling, legal and other services; court accompaniment and in-court support throughout the court process. A Victim Witness Advocate is assigned to a case after the police have found sufficient evidence to pursue criminal prosecution and the case enters the court system. A victim may also go to the court of jurisdiction during court hours and ask to speak to a Victim Witness Advocate. The local police can direct you to the appropriate court and location.

Sample OSHA Citation (Press Releases)

DANBURY HOSPITAL IN DANBURY, CONNECTICUT., was cited by OSHA for failing to provide its employees with adequate safeguards against workplace violence. The OSHA inspection, begun in January 2010 in response to worker complaints, identified several instances during the past 18 months in which employees in the hospital's psychiatric ward, emergency ward, and general medical floors were injured by violent patients. In addition, OSHA noted 25 cases over the past five years in which hospital employees lost workdays or were put on restricted duty after being injured by patients. OSHA found that the hospital's workplace violence program was incomplete and ineffective at preventing these incidents. As a result, OSHA cited the hospital for an alleged serious violation of OSHA's general duty clause for failing to provide a workplace free from recognized hazards likely to cause death or serious injury to workers, in this case the hazard of employees being injured by violent patients. OSHA's citation included suggested means of abatement that the hospital can pursue to reduce workplace violence including:

- Creating a stand-alone written violence prevention program for the entire hospital that includes a hazard/threat assessment, controls and prevention strategies, staff training and education, incident reporting and investigation, and periodic review of the program
- Ensuring that the program addresses specific actions employees should take in the event of an incident and proper reporting procedures
- Ensuring that security staff members trained to deal with aggressive behavior are readily and immediately available to render assistance
- Ensuring that all patients receiving a psychiatric consultation are screened for a potential history of violence
- Using a system that flags a patient's chart any time there is a history or act of violence and training staff to understand the system
- Putting in place administrative controls so that employees are not alone with potentially violent patients in the psychiatric ward

North Suffolk Mental Health Association Inc. was cited and entered into a companywide settlement agreement with the U.S. Department of Labor to implement comprehensive procedures and policies to safeguard its workers better against the hazards of workplace violence. Occupational Safety and Health Administration cited North Suffolk in June 2011 for failing to provide adequate safeguards against workplace violence following the death of a worker in January 2011. A resident of the company's group home in Revere allegedly abducted and murdered the worker, who worked on-site as a senior counselor. North Suffolk contested its citation to the Occupational Safety and Health Review Commission. The settlement, which applies to all North Suffolk programs, activities and workplaces, now resolves the case.

The terms of the settlement include agreeing to a stand-alone written violence prevention program for all client-related service programs at all its locations. The program's elements will include workplace controls and prevention strategies; hazard/threat/security assessments; a workplace violence policy statement outlining, and emphasizing a zero-tolerance policy for workplace violence; incident reporting and investigation; and periodic review of the prevention program. Management will solicit staff input and ensure staff involvement in the workplace violence prevention program, including offering full membership on the company's safety committee.

North Suffolk also agrees to take, at a minimum, the following measures across all its operations, to the extent it hasn't already:

- Implement procedures to communicate any material incident of workplace violence or threatening behavior to staff in a timely manner
- Implement procedures to account for staff who end their shift away from North Suffolk work sites; a buddy system for at least the second and third shifts, as appropriate, based on situational risk assessments; a procedure for staff to request additional coverage when necessary including, but not limited to, situations where staff members communicate that they feel unsafe; and a system for documenting such requests
- Determine the behavioral history of new and transferred clients and utilize a system, such as log books, to identify clients with assaultive or threatening behavior and communicate pertinent information to potentially exposed staff; train staff to understand the system; and have a process in place to respond appropriately to clients who display disruptive behavior
- Provide staff with a reliable way of summoning assistance, such as electronic alarms, cell phones and/or walkie-talkies, when needed on company premises, when staff is alone with a client in the community and/or transporting a client in a vehicle
- Conduct annual risk assessments of each work site to ensure exit routes are available and easily identified. Provide adequate lighting at all company facilities

All workers throughout North Suffolk's operations will be provided with a notice summarizing the settlement, which also advises them how they can easily obtain a copy of the full document.

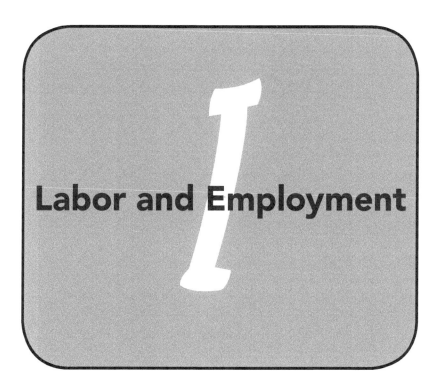

Labor and Employment

HEARING ON SB 483

Maryland Senate Finance Committee
Testimony from Jane Lipscomb, PhD, RN, FAAN

I am writing to provide my strong support for SB483, a performance based law that will reduce workplace violence in healthcare and improve the quality of care delivered. For more than 20 years, I have worked with numerous healthcare organizations across the U.S. to develop programs and policies to reduce workplace violence. This work has supported the passage of state workplace prevention laws in Washington and New York. Over this period of time, I have conducted federally funded research that has demonstrated the feasibility and impact of developing and implementing a comprehensive violence prevention program, similar to that mandated by this bill. I have personally experience the impact that such legislation has, in bringing together workers and healthcare organizations to systematically assess and control the risk of violence to staff and patients alike. The proposed legislation takes a common sense approach to preventing staff injury and improving patient care by requiring the basic elements of any comprehensive health and safety program:

1. An annual comprehensive violence risk assessment and constant recordkeeping
2. Workplace violence prevention committees
3. Annual violence prevention training and education
4. A system for responding to incidents

Opponents to the bill suggest that their segment of the industry should be exempt from coverage by this legislation, in part because of a concern about the stigmatization of the populations they serve. What needs to be emphasized in this hearing is that while acts of aggression and violence in the healthcare environment are often a function of the underlying pathology and unintended by the perpetrator, they are also not deserved by the staff. In addition, exposure to work-related aggression and violence increases the risk of non-therapeutic and negative responses by staff, ultimately leading to diminished quality of care.

As noted in a white paper accompanying this testimony, workplace violence represents a significant threat to the wellbeing of healthcare workers, patient care, and institutional productivity. It also threatens to diminish the overall strength of Maryland's healthcare system at a time of rapid expansion and change—a time when trained, empowered healthcare professionals are more important than ever. The intent of the SB 483 is to create formal mechanisms that will allow management and employees to discuss workplace violence incidents in real-time and create solutions in line with a patient's care plan. At least nine other states have passed laws that mandate workplace violence prevention programs in healthcare facilities. Maryland should do the same to protect our healthcare workforce.

Baltimore Sun Op Ed 2013 (Jane Lipscomb)

WORKPLACE VIOLENCE IS A SERIOUS OCCUPATIONAL HAZARD in hospitals and other healthcare facilities, a fact that has escaped an unsuspecting public. Nationally, nursing assistants employed by nursing homes have the highest incidence of workplace assault among all workers, according to federal data. For women who work in nursing homes, social services and hospitals, the likelihood of being harmed on the job is like that of women working the late-night shift in convenience stores.

To draw attention to these and other hidden risks, the Alliance Against Workplace Violence has designated April as Workplace Violence Awareness Month. On April 28 each year, the unions of the AFL-CIO observe Workers Memorial Day. In Maryland, healthcare and social assistance workers made up just 16% of the state's workforce but accounted for 62% of workplace violence incidents that resulted in at least one day away from work in 2010, the most recent year for which figures are available.

Earlier this year, a broad coalition of stakeholders including workers' unions, the Maryland Hospital Association and advocacy groups came together to address workplace violence in Maryland. The Safe Care Act, legislation that would have strengthened violence prevention at health-care facilities, was introduced in the 2013 General Assembly session but withdrawn after stakeholders representing nursing homes and assisted living facilities strongly opposed the measure. The bill would have improved safety by requiring public and private facilities to establish violence prevention committees consisting of management and employees; establish a violence-prevention program; produce annual violence assessments, and provide regular training for employees.

Workplace Violence Awareness Month calls for greater attention to needed steps such as these. Opponents of the Maryland legislation representing nursing care and assisted living organizations claimed they already have extensive standards and protocols for dealing with work-place violence that are tailored to the individual environments where they care for patients and residents. Not so. Nursing homes in Maryland are required to develop a personal care plan for residents' health and safety, but none to identify and control workers' assault hazards.

I am distressed that the bill was withdrawn. For more than 20 years, I have worked with numerous healthcare organizations across the nation to develop programs and policies to reduce workplace violence. This effort supported the passage of state workplace violence prevention laws in Washington and New York. I have conducted federally funded research that has demonstrated the feasibility and impact of developing and imple-menting a comprehensive violence prevention program, similar to that of the Safe Care Act. Such legislation brings together workers and health-care organizations to systematically assess and control the risk of violence to staff and patients alike. Opponents were also concerned that passage would stigmatize the populations they serve.

The public needs to keep in mind that acts of aggression and violence in the healthcare environment, while unintended by the perpetrators and often due to their underlying pathology or illness, are undeserved by the staff. Exposure to work-related aggression and violence increases the risk of non-therapeutic and negative responses by staff, ultimately leading to diminished quality of care. Although healthcare workers must wait another year to be assured that Maryland's elected officials take their safety seriously, it is everyone's responsibility to hold healthcare facilities accountable. We need to make sure they are safe places to work and receive care.

After all, at one point or another, healthcare facilities are used by all of us. Nothing new would be demanded of any facility that already has put in place a voluntary workplace violence plan that meets the simple criteria in the Safe Care Act. Its common-sense approach to preventing staff injury and improving patient care is one that employers should embrace for the safety of their staffs. The Safe Care Act, or a future bill like it, is further needed to improve institutional productivity and patient care. The lack of such a law could potentially diminish the overall strength of Maryland's healthcare system at a time of rapid expansion and change—a time when trained, empowered healthcare professionals are more important than ever.

At least nine other states have passed laws that require workplace violence prevention programs in healthcare facilities. Maryland, a state recognized for its world-class healthcare institutions, should do the same to protect our healthcare workforce.

Jane Lipscomb is a professor at the University of Maryland School of Nursing. Her email is lipscomb@son.umaryland.edu.

http://www.baltimoresun.com/news/opinion/oped/bs-ed-workplace-safety-20130425-story.html (Published on April 25, 2013).

References

Agency for Healthcare Research and Quality. (2012). Surveys and Tools to Advance Patient-Centered Care. Retrieved from https://cahps.ahrq.gov/quality-improvement/improvement-guide/analysis-of-results/Quantitative-Analyses/Performance-Problems_Tools/Root-Cause-Analysis.html

American Nurses Association. (2012). Position Statement: Reduction of Patient Restraint and Seclusion in Health Care Settings. Retrieved from http://www.nursingworld.org/MainMenuCategories/EthicsStandards/Ethics-Position-Statements/Reduction-of-Patient-Restraint-and-Seclusion-in-Health-Care-Settings.pdf

American Psychiatric Nurses Association. (2008). Workplace Violence: APNA 2008 Position Statement. Retrieved from http://www.apna.org/files/public/APNA_Workplace_Violence_Position_Paper.pdf

APNA. (2014). Position Statement on the Use of Seclusion and Restraint. Retrieved from http://www.apna.org/i4a/pages/index.cfm?pageid=3728

Arnetz, J. E., & Arnetz, B. B. (2001). Violence towards health care staff and possible effects on the quality of patient care. *Social Science Medicine, 52*, 417–427.

Bensley, L., Nelson, N., Kaufman, J., Silverstein, B., Kalat, J., & Shields, J.W. (1997). Injuries due to assaults on psychiatric hospital employees in Washington State. *American Journal of Industrial Medicine. 31*(1), 92–99.

Commonwealth of Massachusetts, Norfolk District Attorney's Office. (2007). *Protecting our Caregivers from Workplace Violence.* Retrieved from http://faculty.uml.edu/jbyrne/44.327/ProtectingOurCaregivers.pdf

Drummond, D. J., Sparr, L. F., & Gordon, G. H. (1989). Hospital violence reduction among high-risk patients. *Journal of American Medical Association, 261*(17), 2531–2534.

ECRI Institute. (2011). *Violence in healthcare facilities.* Healthcare Risk Control - Safety and Security 3, 2. Retrieved from https://www.ecri.org/components/HRC/Pages/SafSec3.aspx

Alexander, B. (2004). Risk factors for work related violence in a healthcare organization. *Injury Prevention, 10*(5), 296–302.

Flannery, Jr., R. B., & Walker, A. P. (2008). Repetitively assaultive psychiatric patients: Fifteen-year analysis of the Assaulted Staff Action Program (ASAP) with implications for emergency services. *International Journal of Emergency Mental Health, 10*(1), 1–8. doi: 10.1007/s11126-010-9152-0.

Friedman, R. (2006). Violence and mental illness—How strong is the link? *New England Journal of Medicine, 355.* doi: 10.1056/NEJMp068229

Harrell, E. (2011). *Workplace violence, 1993–2009: National crime victimization survey and the census of fatal occupational injuries* [Electronic version]. Washington, DC: U.S. Department of Justice.

Hodgson, M. J., Reed, R., Craig, T., Murphy, F., Lehmann, L., Belton, L., & Warren, N. (2004). Violence in Healthcare Facilities: Lessons from the Veterans Health Administration. *Journal of Occupational & Environmental Medicine, 46*(11), 1158–1165.

Hsiang-Chu, P. & Sheuan, L. (2011). Risk factors for workplace violence in clinical registered nurses in Taiwan. *Journal of Clinical Nursing, 20*(9), 1405–1412.

The Joint Commission. (2010). Preventing violence in the health care setting. *Sentinel Event Alert, 45.*

LeBel, J., & Goldstein, R. (2005). The economic cost of using restraint and the value added by restraint reduction or elimination. *Psychiatric Services, 56,* 1109–1114. doi: 10.1176/appi.ps.56.9.1109

Lipscomb, J. A., & Love, C. C. (1992). Violence toward health care workers: An emerging occupational hazard. *AAOHN Journal, 40,* 219–228.

Lipscomb, J. A. (1994). Violence in the health care industry: Greater recognition prompting occupational health and safety interventions. In B. Charney (Ed.), *Essentials of Modern Hospital Safety.* Boca Raton, FL: Lewis CRC Press.

Lipscomb, J., McPhaul, K., Rosen, J., Geiger-Brown, J., Choi, M., Soeken, K., Porter, P. (2006). Violence prevention in the mental health setting: The New York state experience. *Canadian Journal of Nursing Research, 38*(4), 96–117.

Lipscomb, J., Chen, Y., Geiger-Brown, J., Flannery, K., London, M., & McPhaul, K. (2012). Workplace violence prevention in state-run residential addiction treatment centers. *Work: A Journal of Prevention, Assessment & Rehabilitation, 42*(1), 47–56.

May, D. D. & Grubbs, L. M. (2002). The extent, nature, and precipitating factors of nurse assault among three groups of registered nurses in a regional medical center. *Journal of Emergency Nursing, 28*(1), 94-100.

McKenna, K. (2008). *Linking services and safety: Together creating safer places of service.* n.p.: Health Service Executive Ireland. Retrieved from http://www.hse.ie/eng/staff/Resources/hrstrategiesreports/Linking_Service_Safety.pdf

McPhaul, K., Rosen, J., Bobb, S., Okechukwu, C., Geiger-Brown, J., Kauffman, K., Lipscomb, J. (2007). An exploratory study of mandated safety measures for home visiting case managers. *Canadian Journal of Nursing Research, 39*(4), 172–190.

McPhaul, K., London, M., Rosen, J., Murrett, K., Flannery, K., Lipscomb, J. (2008). Environmental evaluation for workplace violence in healthcare and social services. *Journal of Safety Research, 39,* 237–250.

McPhaul, K., Lipscomb, J., & Johnson, J. (2010). Assessing risk for violence on home health visits. *Home Healthcare Nurse, 28*(5), 278–289.

Nachreiner, N. M., Hansen, H. E., Okano, A., Gerberich, S. G., Ryan, A. D., McGovern, M. P., Watt, G. D. (2007). Difference in work-related violence by nurse license type. *Journal of Professional Nursing, 23*(5), 290–300.

National Labor Relations Board. (n.d.). *Protected concerted activity.* Retrieved from http://www.nlrb.gov/rights-we-protect/protected-concerted-activity

New York State Legal Code. (2009).12NYCRR Part 800.8(j)(6)

NIOSH, Centers for Disease Control and Prevention. (1996). *Violence in the workplace.* Current Intelligence Bulletin 57, DHHS (NIOSH) Pub. No. 96-100. Retrieved from http://www.cdc.gov/niosh/docs/96-100/

NIOSH, Centers for Disease Control and Prevention. (2002). Violence Occupational Hazard in Hospitals. Retrieved from http://www.cdc.gov/niosh/docs/2002-101/

Pompeii, L., Dement, J., Schoenfisch, A., Lavery, A., Souder, M., Smith, C., & Lipscomb, H. (2013). Perpetrator, worker and workplace characteristics associated with patient and visitor perpetrated violence (Type II) on hospital workers: A review of the literature and existing occupational injury data. *Journal of Safety Research, 44,* 57–64.

Pompeii, L., Schoenfisch, A., Dement, J., Lipscomb, H., Smith, C. (2014). Contextual factors: What gets reported as workplace violence in hospitals? Paper presented at APHA Annual Meeting: 2014, Nov 15-19, New Orleans, Louisiana.

Pompeii, L., Schoenfisch, A., Lipscomb, H., Dement, J. (2014, Nov). When violence is "part of the job:" Effects on workers, research approaches, and researchers. Paper presented at APHA Annual Meeting, New Orleans, Louisiana.

Quanbeck, C. D., McDermott, B. E., Lam, J., Eisenstark, H., Sokolov, G., & Scott, C. L. (2007). Categorization of aggressive acts committed by chronically assaultive state hospital patients. *Psychiatric Services, 58*(4), 521–528.

Snyder, L. A., Chen, P. Y., & Vacha-Haase, T. (2007). The underreporting gap in aggressive incidents from geriatric patients against certified nursing assistants. *Violence and Victims, 22*(3), 367–379.

U.S. Centers for Disease Control and Prevention, NIOSH. (2002). Violence: Occupational hazard in hospitals. Retrieved from http://www.cdc.gov/niosh/docs/2002-101/pdfs/2002-101.pdf

U. S. Department of Labor, Bureau of Labor Statistics. (2006). *Survey of workplace violence prevention.* Retrieved from http://www.bls.gov/iif/oshwc/osnr0026.pdf

U. S. Department of Labor, Bureau of Labor Statistics. (2012). *Nonfatal occupational injuries and illnesses requiring days away from work, 2011.* USDL-12-2204.

U. S. Department of Labor, Bureau of Labor Statistics. (2013). *Nonfatal occupational injuries and illnesses requiring days away from work, 2012.* USDL-13-2257.

U. S. Department of Labor, Occupational Safety and Health Act of 1970. (1970). Retrieved from https://www.osha.gov/law-regs.html

U. S. Department of Labor, Occupational Safety and Health Administration. (1996). Guidelines for preventing workplace violence for healthcare and social service workers. (No. OSHA 3148), 1996.

U. S. Department of Labor, Occupational Safety and Health Administration. (2004). *Guidelines for preventing workplace violence for healthcare and social service workers.* OSHA 3148-01R.

University of Iowa, Injury Prevention Research Center. (2001). *Workplace violence—A report to the nation.* Retrieved from http://www.public-health.uiowa.edu/iprc/resources/workplace-violence-report.pdf

Welch III, C. E., Hodgson, M. J., & Haberfelde, M. (2012). Impact of medical center complexity on Veterans Health Administration nursing staff incidence rates for reported assaults. *Work, 44*(4), 499–507. doi: 10.3233/WOR-2012-1479.

Wolf, L.A., Delao, A., & Perhats, C. (2014). Nothing changes, nobody cares: Understanding the experience of emergency nurses physically or verbally assaulted while providing care. *Journal of Emergency Nursing, 40*(4), 305-310, doi: 10.1016/i.jen.2013.11.006.

Yragui, N. L., Silverstein, B. A., Foley, M., Johnson, W., & Demsky, C. A. (2012). *The Washington State Psychiatric Hospital Work, Stress, and Health Project: Final report to Washington DSHS Mental Health Division and Western State Hospital.* Unpublished Technical Report.

Index